# THE NEW PHYSICAL FITNESS:

## Exercise for Everybody

By

**Joseph Di Gennaro, Ed.D.**
**Lehman College,**
**Herbert H. Lehman College of**
**City University of New York**

**Morton Publishing Company**
295 West Hampden, Suite 104
Englewood, Colorado 80110

**Printed in the United States of America**

ISBN: 0-89582-097-8

# ACKNOWLEDGMENTS

I wish to express my sincere appreciation and gratitude to:

Jo-Tina DiGennaro, for her valuable recommendations and editorial efforts

Dave Gillison, Dom Totino, and Doug Tsori for their photographic work

All my friends and colleagues at Lehman College for never failing to provide encouragement and help when needed; especially to Kathy Mastriaco, Nick Testa, Blanche Teitelbaum, and Dorothy Campion

My students: Jaquie Moody, Claude Lewis, Pete Batalla, and Evette Bass for their time and effort in taking the photographs

Holt, Rinehart and Winston, Publishers, and M. Evans, Publishers, for permission to use copyrighted materials

And a special word of thanks to the following individuals and companies for their supply of photographs and overall cooperation:

Nautilus Sports / Medical Industries
P.O. Box 1783
Deland, Florida 32720

Universal Gym Equipment, Inc.
930 27th Ave. S.W.
P.O. Box 1270
Cedar Rapids, Iowa 52406.

Jim Bryant
Sports photographer and Professor of Physical Education
Metro State College
Denver, Colorado

# PREFACE

Sometimes I think that my love for physical activity is inherent, because I have performed varying forms of it for as far back as I can remember. As a matter of fact, I have participated in most of the different physical activities that will be discussed in this book, from aerobic dancing to the completion of a 26.2-mile marathon run. My enthusiasm for exercise and physical fitness was greatly reinforced through my formal study of them during my undergraduate and graduate college days. To this very day, I still become excited when I read or listen to reports of the potential values of physical activity, such as the recent one linking regular exercise with the immunity to common bacterial infectious agents. I desire to share with you not only my zeal and fervor for physical activity, but also the most relevant, current concepts and perspectives concerning exercise and physical fitness.

As I wrote this book, I made special effort to present this body of information (which, I might add, grows more voluminous with each passing day) without confusing, baffling, or overwhelming you. Rather, I consciously strived from beginning to end to condense, simplify, and present its contents via interesting discussions written in a conversational tone that all readers could understand and appreciate fully.

The instructional goals of physical education today have advanced quite appropriately from merely making students exercise and taking care of their physical needs temporarily, to more meaningful lifetime behavioral objectives. In line with this new emphasis, my sincere hope is that *The New Physical Fitness: Exercise For Everybody,* will help you to do just that. In short, that it implants and nurtures in each and every one of you the knowledge and competencies requisite to your effectively directing your own physical fitness efforts, as well as enabling you to better experience the joys of exercise for a good many years to come.

Joseph Di Gennaro
New York, New York
1983

# CONTENTS

**Chapter Ten**
### Making Optimal Physical Fitness A Reality: Summary and Conclusions

*For my wife, Jo-Tina;*
*my daughter, Jo-Ann;*
*and my boys, Joe, John, and James*

*"If you give a starving man a fish,*
*he will have enough to eat for one meal;*
*if you teach him how to fish, he*
*will not be hungry for the rest of his life.*

*an old Chinese*
*Proverb*

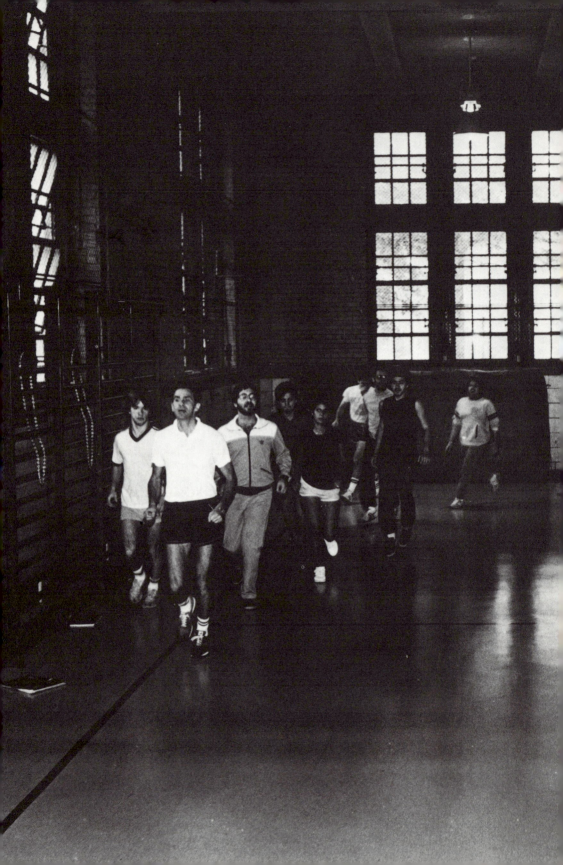

# Chapter One

# INTRODUCTION TO THE STUDY OF EXERCISE AND PHYSICAL FITNESS

*"There is only one subject matter for education, and that is life in all its manifestations."*

Alfred North Whitehead

## HOW MUCH DO YOU KNOW ABOUT EXERCISE AND PHYSICAL FITNESS?

Exercise and physical fitness! Surely you have heard the words a number of times in the past. The owners of health spas springing up in varying localities around the country are spending millions of dollars to advertise their exercise and fitness facilities. As a student in junior or senior high school you were probably given some type of physical fitness test at one time or another. And as a television viewer you might have seen a variety of commercials prepared by the President's Council (on Physical Fitness) urging every American to exercise regularly. Or perhaps you have read one of the articles about exercise and fitness that have been appearing with greater frequency in daily newspapers and popular magazines. Actually, the literature dealing with these topics is not confined to periodicals, because for each year since 1980 some fifty books on physical fitness have been added to the Library of Congress (excluding those dealing with specific physical activities such as walking, jogging, rope-skipping, and swimming).

1

And yet, with all the publicity, fanfare, and dissemination of information regarding it, few have bothered to explain fully the meaning of physical fitness. A universal concept of it continues to elude us. Take a few moments to look up the words in your dictionary. You are going to find that most dictionary compilers fail to render physical fitness definitions at all. Others provide explanations of it that are nebulous and meaningless. Small wonder that most of us tend to conceive of physical fitness so differently; and because of erroneous beliefs, lack of knowledge, and confusion we fail to understand our vital fitness needs as well as how to meet them.

Like countless others, I'm sure you share the general feeling that "exercise is good for you" and that you would like to be "physically fit." Great! But the question is: "Are you capable of guiding your behaviors effectively so as to attain a suitable level of personal physical fitness?" Far too many individuals are currently basing their exercise-fitness actions on popular misconceptions and unfounded premises which abound today, rather than on tested truths, facts, and principles. As a self-check for your knowledge of accepted exercise and physical fitness information, see how well you perform on the quiz that follows.

## EXERCISE-FITNESS SELF-CHECK QUIZ

**Directions:** Read each statement carefully. If you disagree with it, place a check in front of it. (Correct information dealing with each question can be found within the text on the pages noted in the parentheses placed at the end of each statement.)

_____    1.  More Americans engage in regular exercise than do not. (p. 7)

_____    2.  Males need exercise more than females. (p. 81)

_____    3.  Exercise increases appetite. (p. 167)

_____  4. Professional football and baseball players have higher levels of physical fitness than professional ballet dancers. (p. 114)

_____  5. It is good to eat a candy bar for quick energy prior to exercise. (p. 177)

_____  6. City people exercise more than suburban and rural residents. (p. 8)

_____  7. Jogging is the best form of exercise for everyone. (p. 194)

_____  8. Regular exercisers should take vitamin and mineral supplements. (p. 176)

_____  9. You must develop large, bulging muscles to increase their strength and power. (p. 32)

_____  10. The best way to eliminate fat from the buttocks, waist, and thighs is to engage in physical activities that activate these areas. (p. 162)

_____  11. The more one sweats during exercise, the more body weight is permanently lost. (p. 177)

_____  12. Your body returns to its normal resting level of energy expenditure right after you stop exercising. (p. 164)

_____  13. To be of real value, exercise should be painful and exhausting. (p. 87)

_____  14. All people with heart disease should exercise. (p. 83)

_____  15. When attempting to lose weight, eliminate fats completely from your diet. (p. 159)

First of all, did you encounter any difficulty in deciding whether the statements were erroneous or not? And, did you place a check in front of *all* of them? You should have, because to some extent each is fallacious! Although by no means comprehensive in scope, this short quiz should reinforce the premise that much misinformation and a general lack of knowledge (concerning exercise and fitness) exist among many of us.

## WHY THIS BOOK?

This book will present in a logical and clear manner the most relevant, up-to-date information dealing with exercise and physical fitness. The study of its contents should help dispel any false beliefs and should contribute to effective fitness decision-making on your part now and in the future. Hopefully, your level of "exercise-fitness intelligence" should be enhanced. These outcomes seem desirable and timely since modern-day life fosters a host of negative forces that contribute to inactivity and a lack of physical fitness among people throughout the world.

## CONFRONTING YOUR PRESENT EXERCISE — FITNESS BEHAVIORS

Close your eyes, relax, and think a few minutes about where you hope to be in ten years. What might your life responsibilities be at that time? Try to envision your overall body appearance and what level of physical health you will have then. Do you envision regular exercise as being a part of your life-style; and what will be your capacity to perform exercise?

It can be a valuable experience to project into the distant future reflecting upon what we will be like and what our lives might encompass. While not immediately obvious to you now because of the predominant "live for today" philosophy that prevails, current fitness-related habits will be critical in the determination of your bodily appearance, health, ability to handle major duties, and overall quality of life ten and twenty years from today. A major challenge of this text, as I view it, is to influence you to overcome any complacency you may have regarding your future states of health and physical fitness.

I realize that your major concerns and priorities of life are the immediate ones; that is, those that pertain to today, tomorrow, and the week's end at the very latest. Young and old alike from all walks of life seem to have enough difficulty dealing with the unceasing struggles and problems they face daily. Our behaviors are often set in light of "instant pleasure and gratification" with little consideration of their long-range consequences. Understandably so, since the majority of today's youth has grown up with so many threats and stressors (e.g., nuclear war). You might have asked yourself: "Why not live for today because I may not see tomorrow?" Although many people may agree with this reasoning, there is another side to the coin. If one chooses to live day-to-day, why shouldn't each one be the best it can be in all possible ways? Improving one's fitness right now can greatly enhance your health and quality of life today, tomorrow, and, with hopeful optimism, for many years to come. The value of this book (in terms of knowledge acquisition and the nurturing of positive fitness-related values and behaviors) is highly if not completely dependent on the realization and acceptance of a rather basic premise: **Your state of health and fitness, your level of productivity, and your ultimate happiness in ten, twenty, and thirty years are being determined by all of your current behaviors and patterns of living.** And for many of you, it is time to modify those that are potentially harmful and threatening.

## THE STATUS OF EXERCISE AND PHYSICAL FITNESS IN CONTEMPORARY SOCIETY

Would you say that the majority of your fellow Americans show a true concern for physical fitness and engage in suitable exercise on a regular basis? From an observational viewpoint, it certainly appears that the interest in exercise and physical fitness has resurged once again throughout the nation as it has so often in the past. It was back in the 1950s that researchers concluded that fitness levels of children in the United States were inferior to their counterparts in varying localities around the world. This finding induced President Kennedy's creation of the White House Committee on Health and Fitness. J.F.K., a rather enthusiastic exercise-oriented person himself, delegated to the committee the responsibility of formulating and carrying out a program to improve the physical condition of the entire nation. Showing further commitment to this goal, Kennedy wrote a provocative article for the ever-popular *Sports Illustrated* entitled, "The Soft American," in which he stated: "The Greeks knew that intelligence and skill can only function at the peak of their capacity when the body is healthy and strong; that hardy spirits and tough minds usually inhabit sound bodies. In this sense, physical fitness is the basis of all activities in our society, and if our bodies grow soft and inactive, if we fail to encourage physical development and prowess, we will undermine our capacity for thought, for work and for the use of those skills vital to an expanding and complex America."*

During the Sixties a sophisticated approach to the study of exercise and fitness was initiated at many of our institutions of higher learning. College level foundational courses of instruction dealing with this subject matter through lectures, readings, and laboratory work continue to flourish and have even been introduced more recently at the high school level.

--------

*John F. Kennedy, "The Soft American," *Sports Illustrated* (December 1960).

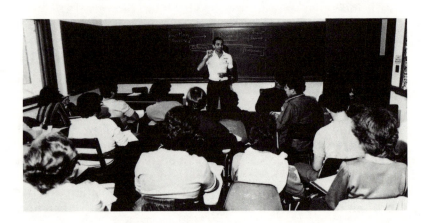

It was also during the 1950s and early 1960s that many prominent authorities in medicine, nutrition, exercise physiology, and psychology began to effectively communicate their enthusiasm for exercise and physical fitness. Continuing through the Seventies and Eighties, more and more professionals have joined the ranks of exercise advocates as the supportive evidence for the potential value of physical fitness continues to mushroom. Over this span of time regular exercise has been implicated in effective weight control and blood fat metabolism, while a lack of physical activity has been associated as a factor in the onset of a variety of threatening chronic debilitators including obesity, circulatory diseases, and backache. The positive functional, structural, and biochemical adaptations that the body can undergo in response to systematic exercise have been reinforced through accepted research findings. And the psychological rewards experienced by the physically active appear to be as relevant during today's hectic times as ever before. In short, a consensus has emerged among prominent health experts throughout the world, that the human requirement for regular exercise is a universal one and as essential to personal health as good food and sleep.

Do not, however, let this discussion mislead you. **Sad as it is to report, the fitness attitudes and habits, the opportunities for exercise, and most alarming of all, the physical condition among the majority of Americans are not what they should be.** Fitness authorities contend that most of our residents lack the awareness of why exercise can be of value to them or how they should go about meeting their fitness needs properly. Current surveys clearly indicate that regular "ongoing, heart pumping" exercise continues to elude two of every three Americans above the age of sixteen.* In a nationwide survey of leisure pursuits among adults, exercise was placed quite low on the list of activities in which they engage. In fact, the number one pastime reported was eating — once again reinforcing the premise that immediate pleasure is a primary behavioral goal among Americans. In descending order of popularity following eating, and placed above exercise on the survey list, were television viewing,

---

*James Cunniff, "Medicine Catches Up with the Sports Boom," *New York Times Magazine* (Section Four), October 5, 1980.
*Jerry Kirshenbaum and Robert Sullivan, "Hold On There, America," *Sports Illustrated*, Feb. 7, 1983.

leisure activity. Thus, the majority of us in this country are failing to meet fitness needs through participation in systematic exercise. Astute observation will confirm this reality. Notice the countless protruding mid-sections among the people you meet each day. Look for, and listen to the frequent reports of aching limbs, sore backs, breathlessness, nausea, and general body discomfort resulting from minimal physical exertion. Consider the number of orthopedic disorders associated with weakened muscles and joints. **In short, a great many of us, our younger generation included, have indeed allowed their levels of physical condition to become horrendously poor.**

In terms of opportunities for exercise, the author is deeply disturbed and concerned by the inadequacies that exist among the poorer, less fortunate segment of our population. In addition to so many other forms of deprivation, these people (most of whom reside in overcrowded urban areas) are being denied ample opportunity to actualize their fitness potentials through joyful physical activity. It might be subtle, but the denial exists. The upper middle-class and affluent residents of surburbia for the most part have access to community swimming, cycling, jogging, gymnasiums, ball playing, racketball, tennis, squash, paddle ball, and country club facilities. Fees for their use when required along with special equipment for participation can be easily afforded. The simple reality for our less fortunate and impoverished population is that when cost is great, the likeli-

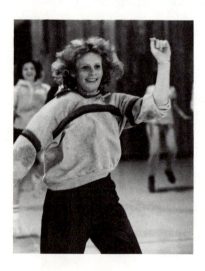
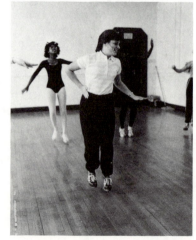

hood of opportunity for healthful physical activity dwindles. And unfortunately, what most large cities provide residents in the way of attractive exercise facilities and supervised fitness programs is quite limited.

Perhaps a day will soon arrive when all people throughout the nation are provided ample facilities and programs to incite their joining the ranks of the physically active. To better prepare for this and help bring it about, each of us would do well to become a serious student of exercise and physical fitness. Let us commence that effort by giving consideration to the extraordinary fitness qualities of the human body that we all too often misuse and abuse.

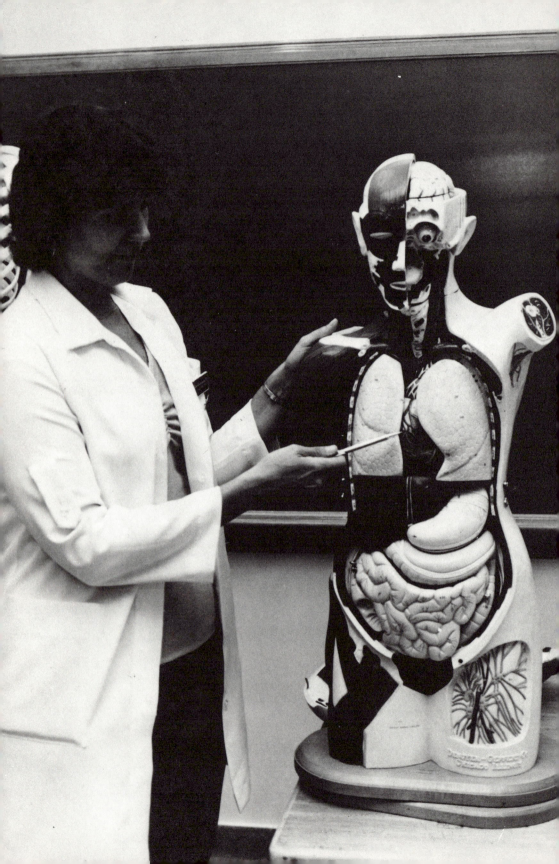

# Chapter Two

# THE INCREDIBLE HUMAN EXERCISE MACHINE

*"What a piece of work is man."*

*William Shakespeare*

---

**KEY WORDS**

| | |
|---|---|
| Exercise | Service Network |
| Metabolism | Aerobic |
| Metabolic Rate | Anaerobic |
| Homeostasis | Regulatory Network |
| Locomotive Network | |

---

## THE MIRACLE OF EXERCISE

"What a piece of work is man." These words of William Shakespeare written centuries ago seem appropriate today, especially when you consider the marvels of the human body. We can easily be misled by the fact that the total cost of all its chemical constituents is only about a dollar. The combining of these substances within the framework of the functioning

11

structure represents an engineering feat of the highest magnitude. The body's modes of operation are so intricate and mysterious, and the roles it serves are so versatile that no amount of money and scientific technology can allow for the fabrication of one human being. Nor has any mechanical structure comparable to it in functional diversity and capacity been devised by man.

The term **exercise** is derived from the Latin *exercere,* which means "to bring about or produce work." **To a great extent, the words human movement, muscular work, physical activity, and exercise are synonymous.** Although inferior to many four-legged animals in balance, speed, and stamina, man, like others in the animal kingdom, was designed for mobility. Further, Homo sapiens has been endowed by his creator with a rather remarkable apparatus that can move through space with relative ease.

I never cease to be amazed and excited by the performances of super athletes, dancers, pianists, circus stars, and others who complete intricate movement feats with extreme precision, timing, grace, style, coordination, agility, and speed. While most spectators admire outstanding movement skills, they seldom give recognition to the covert body operations responsible for the production of them. Consider the level of interaction and organization of internal physiological activity needed to complete a 26-mile marathon or to pound a tennis

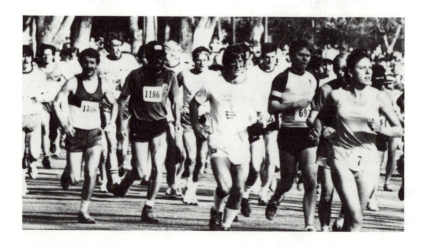

ball over and over again through a variety of strokes and footwork during the course of a three hour tennis match. **During the performance of all physical activities, the body interior takes on the characteristics of a gigantic, computerized chemistry laboratory. The total number of complex biochemical occurrences that initiate and regulate the operation of muscles, bones, and joints; the speeding of blood throughout the body; and the constant communication among sensory organs, the brain, glands, and working organs can stagger the imagination. Yet, the miraculous events associated with the exercise state occur naturally and, at times, without conscious effort.**

# METABOLISM AND HOMEOSTASIS: UNIVERSAL PROPERTIES OF HUMAN LIFE

Your body hosts zillions of basic life units called cells. Certain kinds of them, such as blood cells, are in constant motion. Others (like those that comprise bone) are completely immobile. All, however, are highly dynamic, diversified, and specialized in function. Most cells are microscopic, except for the larger fiber-type cells of skeletal muscle which resemble a human hair in appearance when observed with the naked eye.

Each of the four billion plus human inhabitants of our planet is somewhat unique. Observation indicates that we differ in size, body build, weight, and facial features. Internal structural, biochemical, and functional variations are also likely. Yet, all of us are remarkably similar in that we possess the exact same essential body parts.

Basically speaking, cells of the same kind combine by the millions to form a distinct type of human tissue. A variety of tissues are, in turn, magnificently pieced and woven together into our primary functioning body parts called organs. When several or more organs integrate their operations in carrying out major processes (such as digestion, elimination of wastes, reproduction, breathing, circulation of blood, etc.), we have what is commonly referred to as a body system. Finally, the combined efforts of a network of body systems is requisite to body movement and other major responsibilities associated with the exercise state.

Every cell in your body lives and operates because a countless number of biochemical events occur within its internal compartments. **Metabolism refers to all the complex reactions that are undertaken at the cellular level.** Basically, they can be divided into two major categories: biochemical processes that involve the burning of fuel substances with oxidizing agents for energy production and those incorporated in the subsequent restoration of energy-producing materials. It is energy production that allows cells within body organs to perform specialized functions. In other words, because of the energy released within cells, the heart pumps blood, muscles produce tension, nerves transmit impulses, and glands secrete hormones. Needless to say, metabolic activity is unceasing, taking place even during sleep. **The term metabolic rate implies the degree of total body energy expenditure at a specific time and is most often expressed quantitatively in kilocalories (Kcal.).** (See Chapter 8.)

**In actuality, your body is also constantly striving to maintain a state of equilibrium or balance throughout internal tissue environs — a process called homeostasis.** Interestingly enough, the highest degrees of human metabolism and homeostatic imbalance possible occur during the performance of strenuous exercise. If, at that time, your restorative processes falter, wastes accumulate, cellular operations become limited, energy production dwindles, and your level of exercise performance becomes impaired.

# MAJOR FEATURES OF THE HUMAN EXERCISE MACHINE

As previously implied, the human body can be likened to an exercise machine in that just about every body part in some way contributes to or is affected by the performance of exercise. **There are, however, three major human networks — locomotive, service, and regulatory — whose component systems are most responsible for producing and maintaining the exercise**

**state** (Table 2.1). Let us consider the more important features and characteristics of the vital body parts that comprise each of these machine networks.

### Table 2.1

### Major Body Networks Responsible for the Production and Sustaining of Movement

| Network | Component Parts | |
|---|---|---|
| Locomotive | Bones (Skeletal System) | |
| | Joints (Articular System) | |
| | Muscles (Muscular System) | |
| Service | Heart | |
| | Blood | (Cardiovascular |
| | Blood Vessels | System) |
| | Lungs | (Respiratory |
| | Air Passage Ways | System) |
| Regulatory | Brain | |
| | Spinal Cord | (Nervous System) |
| | Nerves | |
| | Glands (Endocrine System) | |
| | Skin (Integumentary System) | |

## 1. THE LOCOMOTIVE NETWORK

The word "locomotive" implies movement production. Bones, muscles, and joints, which together constitute about 60 percent of total body weight, are primarily responsible for body movements. A highly resilient system of bones not only provides the base of support for the different postures you assume, but is also an effective lever system. Of the 206 skeletal bones that exist, a total of 177 can move through space, allowing for body transportation from place to place and the manipulation of varying objects within its surroundings as well.

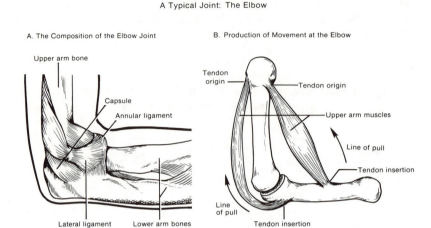

A Typical Joint: The Elbow

A. The Composition of the Elbow Joint

B. Production of Movement at the Elbow

Upper arm bone

Capsule

Annular ligament

Lateral ligament      Lower arm bones

Tendon origin

Tendon origin

Upper arm muscles

Line of pull

Tendon insertion

Line of pull

Tendon insertion

Note: Tendon attachments of two different muscles pull the lower arm bones in different directions.

**Figure 2.1**

Two or more bones meet with each other at junctions called joints. These are the sites where movements of limbs actually take place. Interconnecting bones are often encased within a protective capsule which contains a natural lubricant. Ligaments, which are protective rubber band type cords, hold the bones in place within the joint capsule during their movement.

## MUSCLE MOTORS

Limb movements are produced by the pulling action of muscle tendons. These are cable-like extensions of muscles that link themselves to bones. Skeletal muscles actually originate on various bones and then extend in other directions to eventually insert onto different bones via their tendons. Tension created within the muscle is transferred through its tendon to the bone which is ultimately made to move. Since all movements incorporate this basic process (or slight variations of it), the 650 skeletal muscles of the exercise machine can be regarded as a natural motor system.

Muscle motors, which have Latin names, differ extensively

in size and shape. There are round as well as flat ones. Some are quite long, others short in length. Contrast the miniature muscles located within the inner ear and eye areas, which are only a few millimeters in length, with the sartorius muscle, which can travel as far as two feet across your anterior thigh from the hip to the inner knee.

Muscles cover the skeletal frame in several layers. The major ones comprising the outermost layer are represented in the color insert (page 3).

Long, cylindrical cells are arranged primarily within each muscle motor in clumps or bundles. Yet, each distinct fiber within every bundle has the unique capability to shorten in length (or contract) and to stretch beyond normal resting length.

When thousands of muscle cells contract simultaneously, the entire muscle shortens in its length. We can observe this occurrence as we view the muscle bulging and feel it hardening. Internal tension is created by this process, and it is at once transferred via the tendon to the connecting bone, causing it to move. When relaxation occurs (with the joint returning to its original position), the bulge as well as the tension and hardness within the muscle dissipates. If the joint is made to extend beyond its normal relaxed position, the muscle fibers elongate beyond their normal length, with the total muscle and its tendons also undergoing a state of stretch.

Your muscle motors seldom, if ever, act alone in even the most elementary human movements. Specific muscles generate set movements. Some joints, such as the shoulder, are capable of a variety of movements. Each one of them, while initiated by a different muscle (or group of muscle motors), also brings into action many other local muscles which assume assistance and stabilization responsibilities. Other joints such as your knee joint, on the other hand, are restricted basically to either a forward or backward movement. The two groups of thigh muscles that produce these knee actions work in opposition to each other. In other words, when one bulges and creates tension, the other group is made to stretch in allowing for efficient knee movement. Most major muscle motors for body limbs are arranged and operate in this fashion.

When assuming the upright position, "anti-gravity" muscle motors (joint extensors) contract automatically to keep weight-

**Table 2.2**

**Human Machine Locomotive Network: Specifications**

| Part | Technical Name | Location | Major Features |
|---|---|---|---|
| Movement Levers | Skeletal System | • Extremities<br>• Torso<br>• Neck<br>• Head | • 177 (of 206) utilized in movement.<br>• Strong and resilient.<br>• Protect internal machine parts.<br>• Factory for production of red blood cells.<br>• Storage of vital minerals. |
| Muscle Motors | Skeletal Muscle System | • Originate and insert on varying bones throughout skeletal system | • Largest machine system.<br>• Constitutes 40 percent of machine weight.<br>• Total of 650.<br>• Build up tension to move bones.<br>• Stretch to allow for opposition movement. |
| Lever Joints | Articular System | • Varying localities<br>• Major ones include toes, foot, ankle, knee, shoulder, elbow, wrist, fingers. | • Meet within protective lubricating capsule.<br>• Held within capsule by ligaments. |

bearing joints straight. Among the more significant muscles of the human exercise machine are those of the lower back, which support the spine and the torso, and the abdominal group (or mid-section musculature), which also provides upper body support and allows waist bending. The upper and lower limb musculature, which is among the most powerful within the human body, produces a variety of movements utilized in the performance of popular physical activities. During all human movement, the phenomenal interaction among muscle motors and joints is coordinated by regulatory centers located within the brain and spinal cord.

## 2. THE SERVICE NETWORK

The human exercise machine is equipped with an elaborate network of systems that continuously services all operating parts including those within its locomotive and regulatory apparatuses. Primary service functions include: (1) fuel processing and delivery, (2) oxygen intake and transportation, and (3) waste removal.

### EXERCISE FUELS

The primary energy-producing fuels for muscles are carbohydrate and fat. Fatty acids are broken down within fat cells and are delivered to muscles via the blood. They are utilized in the presence of oxygen (**aerobic**) when the muscle motors are in a resting state and during periods of slight activation or low-intensity exercise. The carbohydrate substance that can be burned either with or without oxygen (**anaerobic**) for a very short period of time is glucose. Glucose and fatty acid are most often used in combination with each other by muscle motors during exercise performance. Protein, while not an energy-producing fuel, is required in the repair and recovery of muscles following their activation.

Food and water are taken into the body periodically. They enter the internal food refinery, the digestive tract (color insert,

## Table 2.3

## Human Machine Fuel Information

| (Energy-Produc-ing) Fuels | When Utilized | Source | Storage Center |
|---|---|---|---|
| Glucose | • Constantly by the brain and spinal cord.<br>• By muscle motors during moderate to heavy exercise. | • Carbohydrate | • Liver<br>• Muscle motors |
| Fat | • By muscle motors at rest and during light to moderate exercise. | • Lipids (fats) | • Body adipose |

p. 6), and are automatically processed into suitable fuel substances which are transferred by the blood to cells for immediate use or to storage tanks where they are housed for future use. The liver and muscle motors themselves serve as fuel tanks for glucose, whereas the major reservoir for fat storage is the machine's fat tissues.

The liver, a blood-cleansing and detoxifying organ, on the average weighs just under four pounds. It is programmed to receive glucose via the blood and to store it until once again needed by muscle motors. It then distributes glucose back into your blood, which again carries it to muscle and nerve centers. A similar cycle of events exists for the conversion and distribution of fatty acids by fat cells, but this takes much longer to occur.

## OXYGEN INTAKE AND PROCESSING

Unlike the case with fuels, there are no oxygen storage tanks within the human exercise machine. Yet, this valuable gas is required constantly by cells throughout the body to burn fuel for energy production. Without a continuous supply of it, our vital organs would fail in their operations and begin to die in a matter of minutes. Thus, the human respiratory system has been designed with specialized parts that provide for ongoing oxygen intake (color insert, p. 5).

Air containing 20-22 percent oxygen is inspired spontaneously through the nose and mouth. It travels downward into a pipe which eventually splits into two major tubes penetrating the lungs. Continuing the journey through an elaborate arrangement of subdividing and progressively narrowing passageways within each lung, the air reaches its final destination — a cluster of tiny sacs. Here, the oxygen present within the air enters readily into blood capillaries, hundreds of which literally encrust each sac. These terminal sacs with their connecting tubular ducts (see color insert, p. 5) resemble a clump of grapes on a vine. Actually, there are hundreds of millions of them in each lung. Carbon dioxide, the gaseous waste carried from internal body tissues by the blood, follows the reverse course of travel to that of oxygen and is thus exhaled from the body.

## FUEL, OXYGEN, AND WASTE TRANSPORT

Blood, blood vessels, and the heart constitute what is commonly called the circulatory (or cardiovascular) system (color insert, p. 4). Its major responsibility is to transport fuels and oxygen to all body organs and to remove wastes formed by their ignition. Biochemically, about 75 percent of the human body is water. Besides the watery fluid present within and surrounding cells, there is that most essential intravascular fluid called blood. It contains and carries nourishing materials to every cell of the body regardless of its location.

In returning from the lungs, blood with dissolved oxygen and processed fuels is pumped by the heart into conductance vessels called arteries. They, in turn, branch out as they travel to all body organs. These arterial branches terminate finally in the tiniest of channels called capillaries, which literally circulate blood throughout the entire organ they penetrate. Here, blood yields oxygen and fuel particles to functioning cells, quickly accomplishes a waste pickup, and continues through the lower portion of the capillary passageway that leads to a system of

**Table 2.4**

## Human Machine Service Network: Specifications

| Part | Technical Name | Location | Major Features |
|------|----------------|----------|----------------|
| Fuel Refinery | Digestive Track | • Internal mid-section | • Constant breakdown and conversion of ingested foods into machine fuels.<br>• Complete digestion in 24 hours.<br>• Removal of solid and liquid wastes.<br>• Process machine fuels into blood for transport to other machine parts. |
| Air Intake and Oxygen Processor | Respiratory Track and Lungs | • Nose, mouth, and down into upper, rear portions of chest cavity | • Process 3-6 liters of air per minute at rest.<br>• Process 80-200 liters of air per minute during exercise.<br>• Contain 600 million air sacs.<br>• Machine's richest capillary supply. |
| Fuel, Oxygen, and Waste Carrier | Blood | • Within internal carrying vessels throughout the machine | • 4-6 liters present.<br>• Carries refined fuels.<br>• Carries .8-1.2 liters $O_2$.<br>• $O_2$ carrying agent is hemoglobin within red blood cells (RBC). |

*(continued)*

# THE HUMAN SYSTEMS

# INDEX

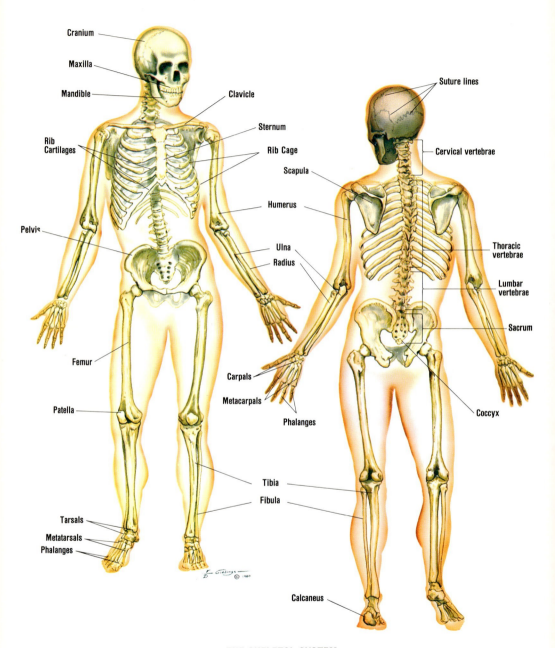

Cranium

Maxilla

Mandible

Clavicle

Sternum

Rib Cartilages

Rib Cage

Pelvis

Femur

Patella

Ulna

Radius

Carpals

Metacarpals

Phalanges

Tibia

Fibula

Tarsals

Metatarsals

Phalanges

Calcaneus

Suture lines

Cervical vertebrae

Scapula

Humerus

Thoracic vertebrae

Lumbar vertebrae

Sacrum

Coccyx

**THE SKELETAL SYSTEM**

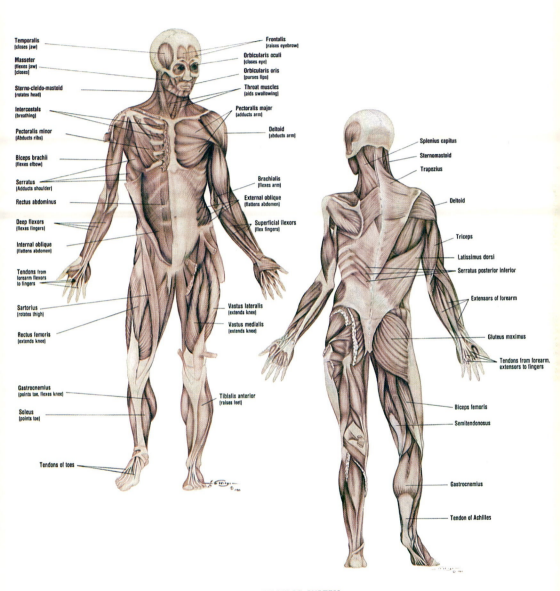

Temporalis
(closes jaw)

Masseter
(flexes jaw)
(closes)

Sterno-cleido-mastoid
(rotates head)

Intercostals
(breathing)

Pectoralis minor
(Abducts ribs)

Biceps brachii
(flexes elbow)

Serratus
(Adducts shoulder)

Rectus abdominus

Deep flexors
(flexes fingers)

Internal oblique
(flattens abdomen)

Tendons from
forearm flexors
to fingers

Sartorius
(rotates thigh)

Rectus femoris
(extends knee)

Gastrocnemius
(points toe, flexes knee)

Soleus
(points toe)

Tendons of toes

Frontalis
(raises eyebrow)

Orbicularis oculi
(closes eye)

Orbicularis oris
(purses lips)

Throat muscles
(aids swallowing)

Pectoralis major
(adducts arm)

Deltoid
(abducts arm)

Brachialis
(flexes arm)

External oblique
(flattens abdomen)

Superficial flexors
(flex fingers)

Vastus lateralis
(extends knee)

Vastus medialis
(extends knee)

Tibialis anterior
(raises feet)

Splenius capitus

Sternomastoid

Trapezius

Deltoid

Triceps

Latissimus dorsi

Serratus posterior inferior

Extensors of forearm

Gluteus maximus

Tendons from forearm,
extensors to fingers

Biceps femoris

Semitendonosus

Gastrocnemius

Tendon of Achilles

## THE MUSCULAR SYSTEM

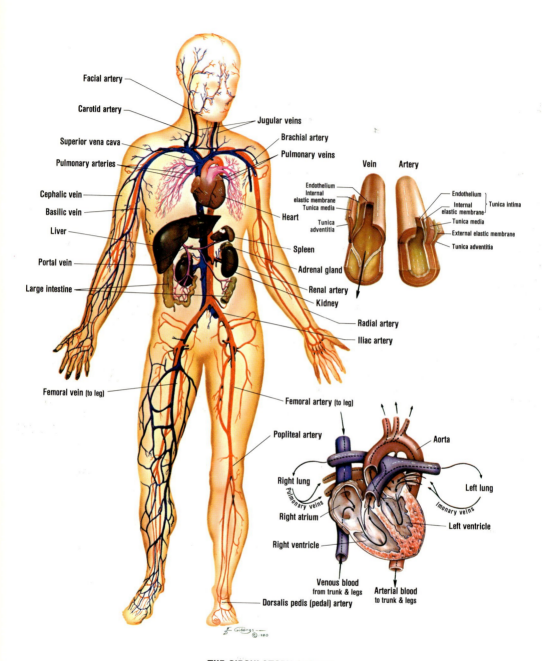

Facial artery

Carotid artery

Superior vena cava

Pulmonary arteries

Cephalic vein

Basilic vein

Liver

Portal vein

Large intestine

Femoral vein (to leg)

Jugular veins

Brachial artery

Pulmonary veins

Heart

Spleen

Adrenal gland

Renal artery

Kidney

Radial artery

Iliac artery

Femoral artery (to leg)

Popliteal artery

Dorsalis pedis (pedal) artery

Vein

Artery

Endothelium
Internal
elastic membrane
Tunica media
Tunica
adventitia

Endothelium
Internal
elastic membrane
Tunica media
External elastic membrane
Tunica adventitia

Tunica intima

Right lung

Pulmonary veins

Right atrium

Right ventricle

Venous blood
from trunk & legs

Aorta

Left lung

Imonary veins

Left ventricle

Arterial blood
to trunk & legs

Giddings
© .980

# THE CIRCULATORY SYSTEM

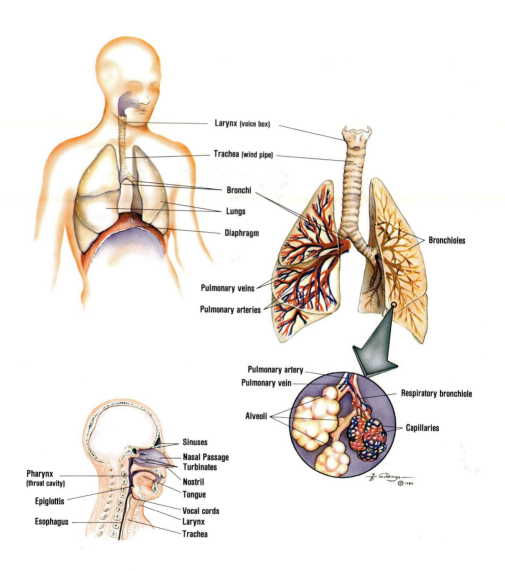

Larynx (voice box)

Trachea (wind pipe)

Bronchi

Lungs

Diaphragm

Bronchioles

Pulmonary veins

Pulmonary arteries

Pulmonary artery
Pulmonary vein

Respiratory bronchiole

Alveoli

Capillaries

Sinuses

Nasal Passage
Turbinates

Pharynx
(throat cavity)

Nostril

Tongue

Epiglottis

Vocal cords

Esophagus

Larynx

Trachea

**THE RESPIRATORY SYSTEM**

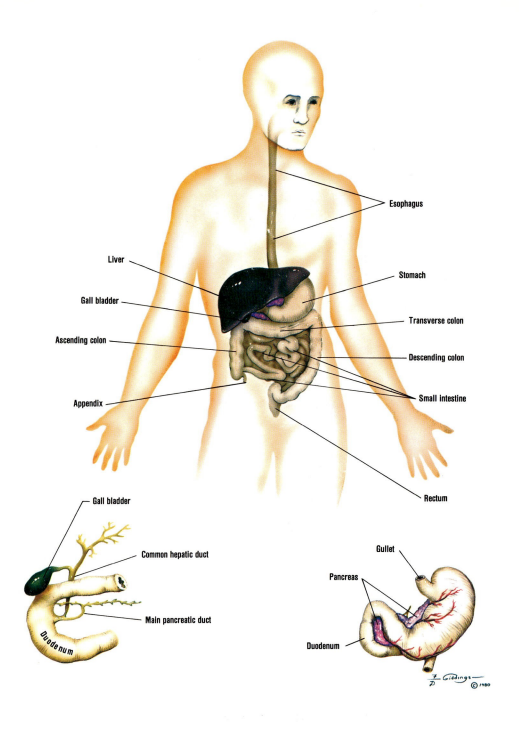

Esophagus

Liver

Gall bladder

Ascending colon

Appendix

Stomach

Transverse colon

Descending colon

Small intestine

Rectum

Gall bladder

Common hepatic duct

Main pancreatic duct

Duodenum

Gullet

Pancreas

Duodenum

F. Giddings
D. © 1980

**THE DIGESTIVE SYSTEM**

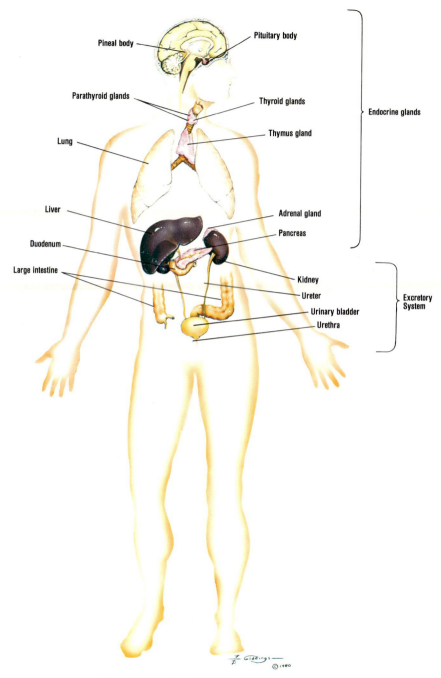

Pineal body

Pituitary body

Parathyroid glands

Thyroid glands

Thymus gland

Lung

Liver

Adrenal gland

Pancreas

Duodenum

Large intestine

Kidney

Ureter

Urinary bladder

Urethra

Endocrine glands

Excretory System

**THE URINARY AND ENDOCRINE SYSTEM**

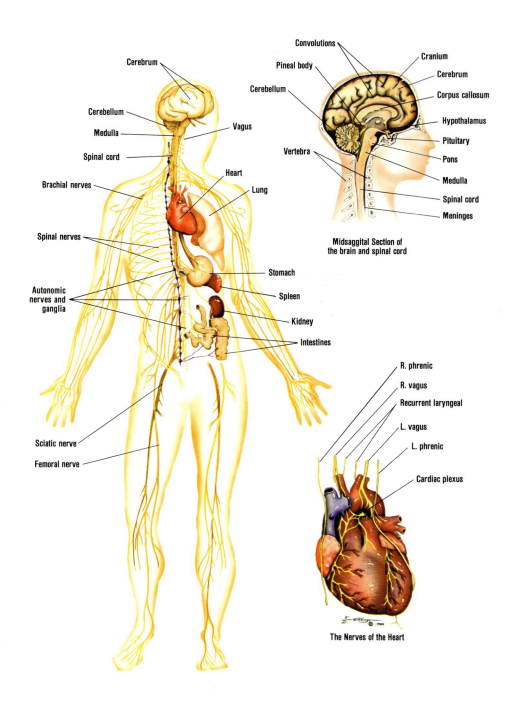

Cerebrum

Cerebellum

Medulla

Spinal cord

Brachial nerves

Spinal nerves

Autonomic
nerves and
ganglia

Sciatic nerve

Femoral nerve

Vagus

Heart

Lung

Stomach

Spleen

Kidney

Intestines

Convolutions

Pineal body

Cerebellum

Vertebra

Cranium

Cerebrum

Corpus callosum

Hypothalamus

Pituitary

Pons

Medulla

Spinal cord

Meninges

**Midsaggital Section of
the brain and spinal cord**

R. phrenic

R. vagus

Recurrent laryngeal

L. vagus

L. phrenic

Cardiac plexus

**The Nerves of the Heart**

## THE NERVOUS SYSTEM

**Table 2.4** (*continued*)

| Part | Technical Name | Location | Major Features |
|------|------|------|------|
| Fuel and O₂ Pump | Heart | ● Center of chest cavity; slightly left of mid-line | ● Can pump 4-6 liters blood per minute. <br> ● Pumps 2,000-4,000 gallons blood per day. <br> ● Rest: Beats about 40-100 times per minute. Exercise: Can beat as rapidly as 200 times per minute. |
| Blood Carrier Vessels | Vascular System: (arteries, veins, and capillaries) | ● Throughout machine from skin to all internal parts | ● Over 60,000 miles in length if laid out in straight line. |

return pathways to the heart called veins. Incredibly, the complete nutrient-waste exchange process at the capillary level occupies a mere second or two.

## THE BLOOD PUMP

The human exercise machine's blood pump is the heart. It is a most amazing device that sustains life by continuously propelling blood to all body localities.

Weighing less than a pound and about the size of the fist, the action of a well-constructed, efficient heart pump is potentially powerful and tireless. In actuality, it is a double pump, one of which constitutes its right side and the other its left. The right and left pumps are separated by a solid wall of tissue. Each distinct pump is composed of a thinly walled blood reception compartment called an atrium and by a blood ejection compartment called a ventricle. The ventricle is constructed with thick walls, more so on the left side of the heart than on the right, since the left ventricle is responsible for pumping blood into the machine's arterial network.

# 3. THE REGULATORY NETWORK

## COMPUTER AND ELECTRICAL WIRING NETWORK

A high degree of regulatory activity within your service and locomotive networks is provided by the 200 billion plus cellular units that comprise your computer center and the system of electrical wires that connect to them (and all other functioning body parts). Imagine! These control mechanisms are so vast and sophisticated that their actual mode of operation continues to baffle the most intelligent of neurophysiologists. Different areas within the main control center, a computer-like structure we call the brain, constantly direct and guide our muscle motors, lungs, blood vessels, and heart pump. Perhaps the single most complicated piece of matter within the entire universe, this master body regulator hosts billions of nerve cells which interconnect among themselves at trillions of sites. In so doing, the brain is potentially capable of storing 200 billion separate bits of information. The jelly-like mass of tissues that constitutes the brain is encased within a bony protective covering (the skull). Although it weighs a mere three pounds or so, a mechanical computer of equal capacity to the human brain would no doubt be larger than both buildings of New York City's World Trade Center put together.

Nerve impulses are directive messages that travel to and from the brain through a rather intricate and elaborate electrical wiring system (color insert, p. 8). The extension of the brain at its base is called the spinal cord (which attaches to its base). The nerve impulses also exit from varying segments of this cord as it travels down the back within a protective bone encasement, the spinal column.

Nerves which emanate from the brain directly or from segments of the spinal cord consist of thousands of compacted bundles of fiber extensions of nerve cells.* Each fiber travels to a predetermined body organ terminating in anywhere from a few to several thousand distinct contact endings. In a muscle

---

*The nerve cell is called a neuron. The fiber portion of it that travels from its central body can vary in length from a few millimeters to six feet.

motor, each microscopic terminal nerve ending contacts with a separate muscle fiber. Any muscle lacking a properly functioning wiring setup will be incapable of undergoing the shortening process.

During exercise, a fantastic array of spontaneous electrical responses occurs within the brain, spinal cord, and peripheral nerves. To simplify these complex happenings, it could be said that hundreds of thousands of nerve impulses are initiated, relayed, and weighed instantaneously within regulatory devices. The end result is the projection of a series of signals carried to varying muscle motors instructing them of when and how much tension to produce in the performance of the desired limb movement. Simultaneously, directives are also channeled to service and other regulatory machine parts including the glands, skin, heart, and blood vessels — thus altering their operations to accommodate the elevated demands for oxygen and fuel.

## BIOCHEMICAL REGULATORS

Endocrine glands, located in varying body areas, produce important biochemical substances called hormones (color insert, p. 7). They are secreted into the bloodstream and make their way to the cells of the body. Hormones promote an internal biochemical balance within organs and promote cellular repair and growth. Without them most organic functions, including the combustion of fuels within muscle motors, would either be severely handicapped or cease entirely.

## BODY TEMPERATURE CONTROL

The skin, consisting of a thin outside layer and a thicker inside one, is seldom thought of as a human organ. Yet, this large, complex structure that covers the entire periphery of the body performs critical life-sustaining functions. It not only hinders the invasion of contaminating agents from entry into the body, but it also provides a system of temperature control. Heat produced by combustive reactions occurring throughout internal body parts is transferred via the circulating blood to tiny conductance vessels located within the inner skin layer. During exercise, these vessels are made to expand (through

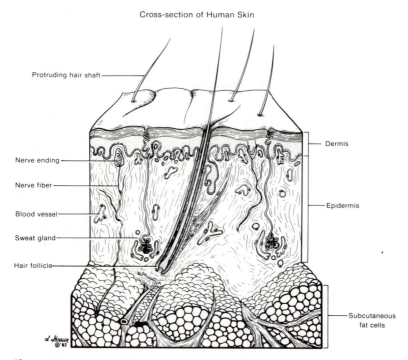

Cross-section of Human Skin

Protruding hair shaft

Dermis

Nerve ending

Nerve fiber

Epidermis

Blood vessel

Sweat gland

Hair follicle

Subcutaneous fat cells

**Figure 2.2**

nervous regulation) in order to receive larger volumes of heated blood. The heat buildup obviously results from intensified metabolism associated with repetitive muscle contractions. Tiny sweat glands within the skin are also activated to allow for the production of perspiration, the evaporation of which induces the dissipation of heat from the blood. When the exercise is curtailed and the temperature of the blood falls, perspiration ceases, and heat is contained rather than given off to the environment. Proper regulation of temperature and fluid levels is essential to continued operational efficiency of the body during both exercise and rest, but more about this later. Let us first proceed to enhance our comprehension of the nature of physical fitness.

**Table 2.5**

# Human Machine Regulatory Network: Specifications

| Part | Technical Name | Location | Major Features |
|------|---------------|----------|----------------|
| Computer Center | Brain | • Within skull bones. | • Pinkish-grey color.<br>• Weighs about 3 pounds.<br>• Composed of over 20 billion nerve cells packed in supportive tissue.<br>• Varying parts direct and coordinate all machine functions.<br>• Cerebral cortex controls muscle motors. |
| Main Extension Cord | Spinal Cord | • Connects to lower brain and travels down spinal column from neck to lower back. | • Elongated cord of nerve tissue.<br>• About width of a pencil.<br>• Contains tracts that carry information and directions to and from brain and machine parts. |
| Electrical Regulatory Wires | Nerves (Spinal and Cranial)<br><br>Tracts (Spinal Cord and Brain) | • Emanate from brain and segments of spinal cord.<br>Within brain and spinal cord. | • 12 pr. of cranial nerves that direct heart pump, lungs, facial muscle motors and other internal machine parts.<br>• 31 pair of spinal nerves that direct muscle motors of limbs and torso. |

*(continued)*

**Table 2.5** (*continued*)

| Part | Technical Name | Location | Major Features |
|---|---|---|---|
| Bio-Chemical Messenger Producers | Endocrine Glands (System) | • Within brain, neck, internal mid-section, and reproductive organs. | • Complex machine parts that secrete important chemical regulators that influence many machine functions. |
| Machine Temperature Regulator | Skin (Integumentary System) | • Envelops entire periphery of the body. | • 18 square feet if laid out. <br> • Protects internal machine parts from harmful chemicals and biologic agents. <br> • Temperature control device. <br> • One square inch contains one yard of blood vessels, 4 yards of nerve receptors, 100-200 sweat glands, and 300 million cells. |

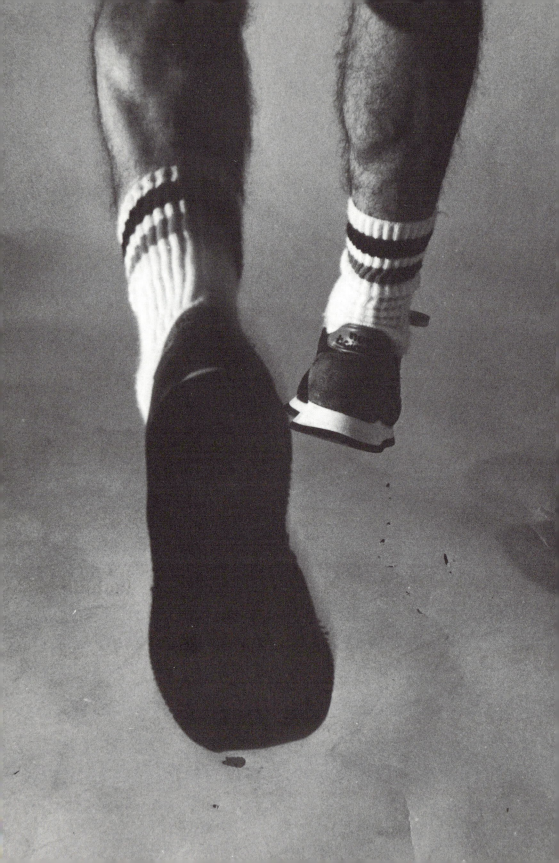

## Chapter Three

# DIMENSIONS OF PHYSICAL FITNESS: CURRENT PERSPECTIVES

*"In strenuous exercise, the demands for oxygen are greatly increased, and the tireless (heart) pump responds accordingly. The heart of a trained athlete in action may pump over 30 quarts of blood per minute — enough blood to carry fifteen times as much oxygen from his lungs. This superior oxygen-capturing power distinguishes the trained man.*

Arthur Steinhaus

---

**KEY WORDS**

| | |
|---|---|
| Physical Fitness | Aerobic Exercise |
| Body Leanness | Anaerobic Exercise |
| Obesity | Steady State |
| Service Network Efficiency | Strength |
| Adiposecyte | Endurance |
| Overeating | Flexibility |
| Heart Rate | Optimal Physical Fitness |

# THE COMPONENTS OF PHYSICAL FITNESS

Physical fitness, a term that is difficult to define, has implied different meanings to people over the years. Not too long ago, the "Charles Atlas" body build was the accepted symbol of fitness. Now, it is evident to most authorities that being physically fit involves a great deal more than just having large muscles and a shapely physique. Having considered the body systems utilized in exercise, you should recognize that **physical fitness is a dynamic state of being, characterized by three integrated components: body leanness, service network efficiency, and locomotive network efficiency.** The discussions that follow will enhance your comprehension and appreciation of the nature of physical fitness.

# BODY LEANNESS

Most students fail to realize that leanness is an integral component of physical fitness. Such a body state is characterized by the dominance of lean tissues as opposed to fat (adipose) tissue. **Obesity, a term signifying a condition in which the body is burdened with excessive adipose,** is the opposite of body leanness.

It was reported previously that one of the primary sources for food storage within the body is the fat cells, or **adiposecytes.** All of us have them but, obviously, some people have more than others. There are varying periods in life when adipose cellularity, the creation of adiposecytes, occurs. The major times seem to be during pre-birth, ages zero to two, and adolescence. Thus, the foundation for one's obesity could have been set quite some time ago. Unfortunately, the nature of adipose tissue is such that once an obesity problem is created, it tends to remain for a lifetime. For one thing, the adiposecyte has a greater propensity for growth than any other kind of body cell. It can expand extensively, like a sponge, to absorb digested food after entry through its cell walls. When a person does bring

Comparison of Normal and Enlarged Adiposecytes

A. Adiposecytes of Normal Size:
   Greater Potential for Body Leanness

B. Enlarged Adiposecytes:
   Greater Potential for Obesity

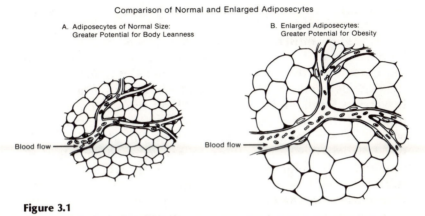

Figure 3.1

about a reduction in body fat, the total number of adiposecytes actually remains the same, despite their shrinkage in size. In other words, once formed, fat cells cannot be eliminated. Rather, they remain in body areas where developed, ever prone to hypertrophy (size increase). This reality could very well be the basis for the "roller coaster" pattern of weight reduction in many chronically obese people, whereby they alternately lose pounds through some popular weight reduction plan and then gradually regain them when the prescription is shelved.

When adipose cellularity takes place, fat tissue accumulates both internally and subcutaneously (just below the skin). The external fat tends to settle mainly within the membranes covering the stomach and intestines* as well as over the musculature of the backside, hips, and upper arm and leg areas where it is most often noticeable. This outer layer of fat, in addition to the provision of food storage, allows for insulation against the cold and the protection of internal organs. However, adiposecytes are basically inert (metabolically inactive) and unlike muscle cells, they are incapable of energy production at rest. For this reason, a 160-pound obese person will expend less energy

---

*Flab in this area can contribute to back problems. By increasing the weight the spine must support, it adds to the pressure of vertebral disks. It can also lead to the protrusion of the visceral organs into the abdominal wall, thus exaggerating the curve of the lower back.

during periods of rest than will a lean individual of the exact same body weight.

Since they must be supplied with nutrients contained in the blood, stores of fat have a tendency to interfere with the performance of the service network. The heart is burdened by the extra demands for blood made of it by excessive fat present in varying localities of the body. Blood transferred to large masses of inert adipose is blood diverted from metabolically active tissues in need of vital nourishment. The addition of body weight from extra fat intensifies the energy requirements of all required and voluntary physical activities, while especially stressing weight-bearing bones, muscles, and joints. Evidently, they must work harder in supporting and transporting the excess body fat. Obese persons are, therefore, more likely to suffer fatigue and injury as results of exercise performance.

It has been established through research findings that obesity is associated with reduced longevity and that the greater the degree of it, the shorter the potential length of life. Statistical studies to date also indicate that obese populations have a higher incidence of the most serious chronic health disorders including high blood pressure, heart disease, stroke, cirrhosis of the liver, diabetes, nephritis, gall stones, backache,

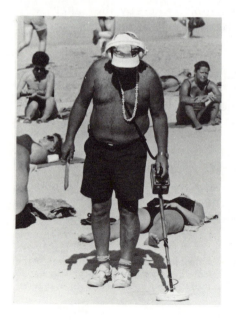

Remember that the "shape" you are in today will determine your "shape" in five, ten, and twenty years.

## Table 3.1

## Summary of the Relevant Features of Body Leanness

- Linked to increased longevity.
- Associated with higher potential of health and prevention of many chronic ailments including cardiovascular diseases.
- Less risk in surgery than obese.
- Positive factor in exercise performance: less energy expenditure, reduced fatigue, less prone to injury.
- Less stress to spine and reduced tendency to suffer backache.
- Higher personal regard for self and greater potential for positive self-concept.
- Better physical appearance.

and even certain cancers. Finally, an obese individual has more complications when undergoing and recovering from surgery than his lean counterpart. Are these grounds enough for considering body leanness as a high priority component of health and physical fitness?

While impossible to determine the number precisely, **it can be estimated that some 50 to 80 million of us suffer some degree of obesity.** (The procedures for evaluation of body leanness in Chapter 4 will help you to determine if you might be one of them!) How and why has it been possible for as much as 35 percent of the U.S. population to have become and to remain obese? Obviously, a great deal of ignorance and apathy exist concerning both the extent and dangers of the problem. Yet, the major reason for its rather high prevalence lies in science's failure to provide adequate answers regarding both the etiology (causation) of obesity and effective remedies for it. Authorities in medicine and nutrition have ascertained that with relatively few exceptions **"overeating," the consumption of more food than the body needs, is the major causative agent for obesity.** They are also well aware of the fact that overeating can result from the failure to burn normal amounts of energy due to extreme physical inactivity as well as from excessive appetite.* What remains a puzzle, despite extensive scientific inquiry, is why so many people eat too much and/or are sedentary in their daily life-styles. Equally baffling is the discovery of a truly effective plan of attack to aid people in reversing behaviors that contribute to their overeating. This dilemma is quite similar to the one posed by the disease of alcoholism. The problem persists not merely because of the existence of alcoholic beverages, but more so because of unidentified physiological and psychological inadequacies that make the alcoholic dependent on the use of these beverages.

Is there any hope for effective obesity control? Yes there is — especially among those with slight to moderate problems. These individuals can join and remain permanently within the ranks of the lean by following the ameliorative plan of action presented in Chapter 8.

# SERVICE NETWORK EFFICIENCY

This author believes that the most relevant component of physical fitness is the operational effectiveness of the service network, more technically referred to as **cardiovascular-respiratory fitness and aerobic efficiency.**\*\* It is also thought of in everyday terminology as body **stamina, wind, and endurance.**

Exercise physiologists contend that the major factor influencing cardiovascular-respiratory fitness is the heart's capacity to pump blood, which ultimately depends on the strength of its muscular walls. Obviously, the more powerful these walls, the greater the degree of force exerted in each heartbeat and the larger the potential volume of blood ejected by it. If the heart is functioning efficiently, it could pump 20-30 liters\*\*\* of blood

---

*Appetite, which is the desire or craving for food, will often exist in the absence of hunger, which is more of a physiological need for food.

\*\*Aerobic efficiency will be the term used most often in subsequent references to this component of fitness.

\*\*\*A liter is a metric measure that is equal to 1.06 quarts.

per minute during exercise. Contrast that to an unconditioned, inefficient one which might be capable of a maximum output of only some six liters of blood per minute.

Air intake and circulatory processes, as might be expected, also contribute to aerobic efficiency, In fact, blood which transfers more oxygen to activated muscles during exercise makes its way to and from the heart and working muscle tissues in a matter of 15-20 seconds. There is also a significant redistribution of blood that occurs during exercise. The blood in the body is actually diverted from certain body organs (mainly within the digestive system) to active muscles where blood vessels open more fully to receive it.

Recall that when you perform physical activity, nutrients and oxygen must be supplied readily to active locomotive and regulatory organs to meet their elevated metabolic demands. Without these materials, increased levels of energy production would be impossible to sustain. Thus, the movements of the physical activity would be curtailed.

**In sum, a strong heart combined with efficient air intake and blood transmission mechanisms (provided via smooth operations carried out within the lungs, blood vessels, and blood) guarantee the delivery of the metabolic materials essential to the maintenance of an exercise state.** Conversely, cardiovascular and respiratory limitations can only lead to partial or complete cessation of energy production within activated locomotive organs, resulting in a reduced ability to perform many forms of exercise.

## ANAEROBIC AND AEROBIC EXERCISE

Skeletal muscle cells are unique in that they function without oxygen for relatively short time periods. The performance of activity without adequate free oxygen is called **anaerobic exercise.** An oxygen deficit within the body is created during anaerobic exercise, since the oxygen required by working muscles exceeds that which is available for consumption. Obviously, the wider this difference in required and available oxygen, the greater will be the oxygen deficit and the production of the harmful waste product, lactic acid. Naturally, this oxygen difference must be made up after anaerobic physical

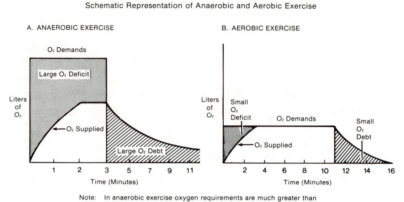

Schematic Representation of Anaerobic and Aerobic Exercise

A. ANAEROBIC EXERCISE                                    B. AEROBIC EXERCISE

Note:    In anaerobic exercise oxygen requirements are much greater than
         in aerobic exercise. Oxygen cannot be supplied to meet demands for
         it and a large oxygen deficit (lactic acid) accumulates. Exercise ceases
         in a matter of minutes after which a rather large $O_2$ debt must be repaid.
         In aerobic exercise adequate oxygen is supplied to meet requirements.
         Exercise can be continued for 10 minutes or longer. Oxygen deficit and
         debts are relatively small.

**Figure 3.2**

activity ceases. The amount of oxygen repaid to the body during
the recovery period is called oxygen debt. Actually, the capacity
to execute anaerobic exercise tasks varies among individuals. It
is, however, quite limited in everyone due to the pain and
discomfort associated with the accumulation of lactic acid and
other physiologic conditions produced by the extreme metabolic demands of the anaerobic state. For example, one cannot
run at maximum speed (a highly anaerobic exercise task) for as
long as she or he can walk, a task which is generally not
anaerobic and does not result in rapid oxygen utilization. (See
Figure 3.2)

   If the level of oxygen required by activated muscles does
not exceed the volume of oxygen being supplied, the individual
is engaged in **aerobic exercise.** The service organs can easily
deliver adequate oxygen to burn fuels that produce energy for
muscle contraction when the metabolic demands of exercise
are not excessive. Thus, in aerobic exercise, there is neither an
extensive oxygen deficit nor a lactic acid accumulation (Figure
3.2).

# THE RELEVANCE OF HEART RATE IN "STEADY STATE" EXERCISE

Physical activity sustained at a steady or even rate for three minutes or more is called **"steady state"** (continuous) exercise. Here the **heart rate, the number of times the heart beats or pumps per minute,** rises to a specific level and remains relatively static due to the constant pace of energy production. Steady-state heart rate is a valuable piece of information that indicates: (a) the degree of stress or demand produced by exercise, and (b) the relative level of aerobic efficiency. Let's say that someone performs three different steady-state exercise tasks (X, Y, and Z) for ten minutes on separate occasions. For task X the steady-state heart rate is 100; while for task Y it is 150; and for

**Figure 3.3**

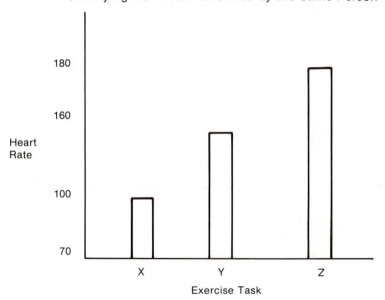

Steady State Heart Rates from Three Exercise Tasks of Varying Demands Performed by the Same Person

Note:   Exercise task X is easy and demands are slight. Task Y is more difficult to perform and demands are moderate. Exercise task Z is the hardest to perform and the demands are quite heavy.

task Z it is 160. This information clearly indicates that Z was the most strenuous of the exercise tasks.

It should be emphasized that the degree of demand produced by exercise (as well as the fitness capacity to meet those demands) will vary quite widely among different individuals. For example, while an exercise task of a set energy output (produced under controlled laboratory conditions) might be performed quite easily at a steady heart rate of 130 by a highly fit person, the same exact task might cause the heart rate of an unfit person to climb to 180. In the latter case, the subject would be forced to utilize anaerobic energy production mechanisms, resulting in oxygen deficit and lactic acid accumulations and, finally, exhaustion. This would not be true for the former subject whose steady-state heart rate of 130 is indicative of a high level of aerobic efficiency and, thus, the production of

**Figure 3.4**

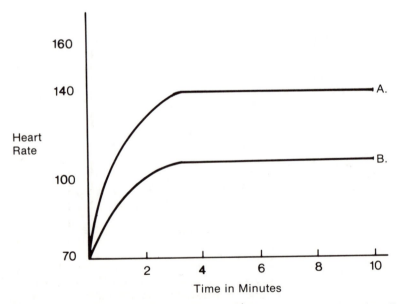

Steady State Heart Rate Responses to the Same Exercise Task in Fit and Unfit Persons (A and B)

Note: Can you explain why B has the more functionally efficient service network?

energy within activated muscles mainly through aerobic mechanisms.

**In sum, the more effective the operational efficiency throughout the service network, the greater the capacity of the body to sustain high energy expenditure exercise. The person with aerobic fitness will perform it with less effort and without tiring quickly.** Since aerobic efficiency also reflects to some degree the health status of the cardiovascular-respiratory organs, exercise stress tests are being more widely used for such appraisals in the field of medicine.

# LOCOMOTIVE NETWORK EFFICIENCY

A person with a quality network of bones, joints, and

**Table 3.3**

**Major Characteristics of Locomotive Network Efficiency**

| | | |
|---|---|---|
| | • Strength: | The maximum force or tension a muscle motor can exert in lifting, pulling, or pushing a resistance. |
| **Skeletal** **Muscles** | • Power: | (A form of strength, but with the time factor added.) The ability of a muscle motor to build up tension quickly. |
| | • Endurance: | The ability of muscle motors to continue in operation for long time periods. |
| **Bones** **and** **Joints** | • Stability: | The capacity of bones and joints to resist the stress of forceful movements. |
| | • Flexibility: | The ability of a joint to move through full range of motion. (Although a characteristic of the joint, it is determined, in part, by stretch ability of muscle and tendon.) |

skeletal muscles will be more capable of exercise performance and less prone to potentially damaging effects of stress placed upon them. The major features indicative of locomotive efficiency include **strength, power, endurance, stability, and flexibility** (Table 3.3).

Obviously, these characteristics differ in varying localities of the body. Proper posture and body carriage, as well as the resistance to debilitating injury and muscle-joint stiffness and soreness, are fostered when minimal levels of efficiency exist within the more significant parts of the locomotive network (back, mid-section, and weight-bearing aspects of the lower extremity).

---

# OPTIMAL PHYSICAL FITNESS

---

Are superior fitness capacities innate or acquired during the course of a lifetime? This is a relevant question which cannot be simply answered by the choice of either alternative. **In reality, it could be concluded that a host of factors relating to age, heredity, environment, and behavior will interact to produce one's ultimate physical fitness status.**

Our "blueprint" for physical health and fitness was supplied by heredity. Every one of us begins life with certain structural, morphologic, and functional potentialities that were determined genetically. Body shape; proneness to obesity; bone structure; size and condition of the heart, lungs, and visceral organs; and total number of cells within skeletal muscles were actually fixed at birth. It can rightfully be said that some of us have a constitutional predisposition to a high level of fitness, while others do not. Evidently, it is not within an individual's power to control genetic makeup. Nor can chronologic age be altered. Actually, all human beings reach their greatest physiological potentials for physical fitness between the ages of 18 and 25. Then, with the passage of time and our getting older in years, the potentiality recedes gradually.

Major environmental determinants of fitness (such as where we live and work) can sometimes be changed; other times, they cannot. However, a lack of control over any influ-

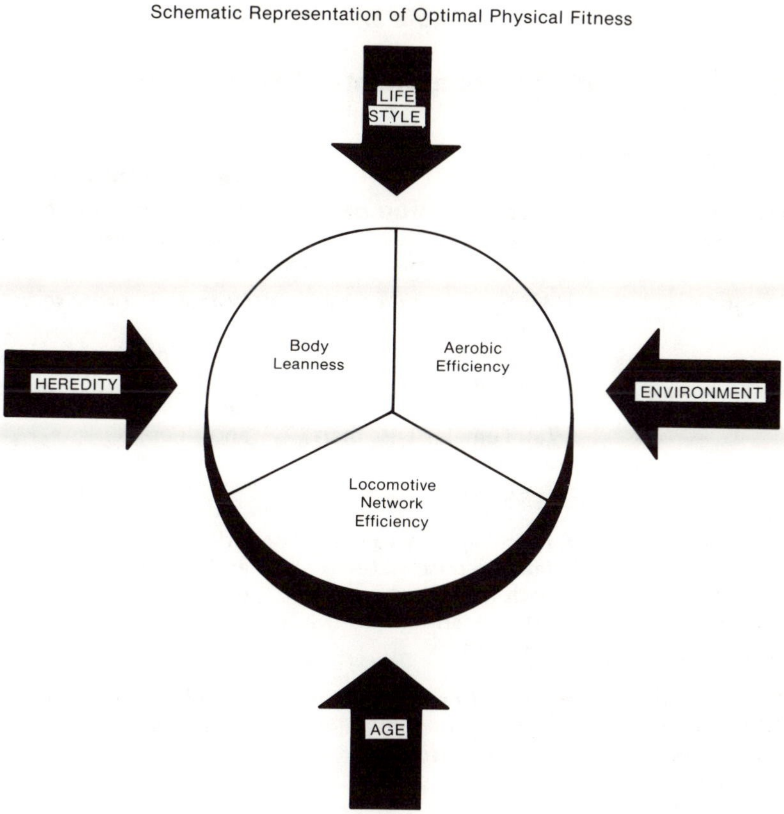

Schematic Representation of Optimal Physical Fitness

**Figure 3.5**

encing fitness factor is not intended to imply that one should be fatalistic and regard personal efforts to enhance fitness as being futile. **Positive behavior patterns associated with proper nutrition, exercise, rest, relaxation, and sleep along with the avoidance of excessive stress and ingestion of harmful substances into the body can often offset the degree of influence of many uncontrolled forces that contribute to excessive body fat, inefficient service network mechanisms, and muscular-joint weaknesses.**

Åstrand, a world-renowned exercise physiologist, believes that the dimensions and functions of aerobic efficiency can be favorably influenced by suitable exercise, especially during the early childhood through adolescent years when body growth

## Table 3.4

## Summary of the Components of Physical Fitness

| Fitness Component | Manifestation of Fitness Component | Keys to Optimal Development and Maintenance |
|---|---|---|
| Leanness | • Absence of excessive body fat.<br>• Standards: Males-Less than 19% of body weight being fat. Females-Less than 22% of weight being body fat. | • Systematic exercise.<br>• Proper nutrition.<br>• Rest, relaxation, and sleep. |
| Aerobic Efficiency | • High capacity to sustain exercise states with less effort, fatigue, and quicker recovery. | • Adequate recovery and repair following exercise. |
| Locomotive Network Efficiency (Strength, Power, Endurance, Stability, and Flexibility) | • Normal posture — no deformity, stiffness, and pain from weakness.<br>• High capacity of locomotive parts to perform and recover from stressful movements without disability and infirmity. | • Avoid abusive habits (smoking, alcohol, drugs). |

and development occur.* Constructive fitness measures may not cancel limiting genetic, environmental, and aging forces completely, but they will most assuredly produce **optimal physical fitness. This is the highest status of physical fitness that can be achieved by each one of you.**

---

*Astrand and K. Rodahl, *Textbook of Work Physiology* (New York: McGraw-Hill Book Company, 1977).

The hallmarks of modern-day living — constant stress, too little rest and relaxation, infrequent (sporadic) or no recreational exercise, overeating, consumption of poor quality foods, and excessive ingestion of cigarette smoke, alcohol, and hard drugs — can only deteriorate health. Further, they will also gradually reduce each component of fitness to a subminimal level even among those of us with positive constitutional make-ups. A life-style characterized by positive fitness behaviors, on the other hand, can only serve to favorably modify fitness. Chapters 5 through 10 will help you to identify those behaviors, but prior to that, our efforts will be directed toward the appraisal of our current physical fitness status.

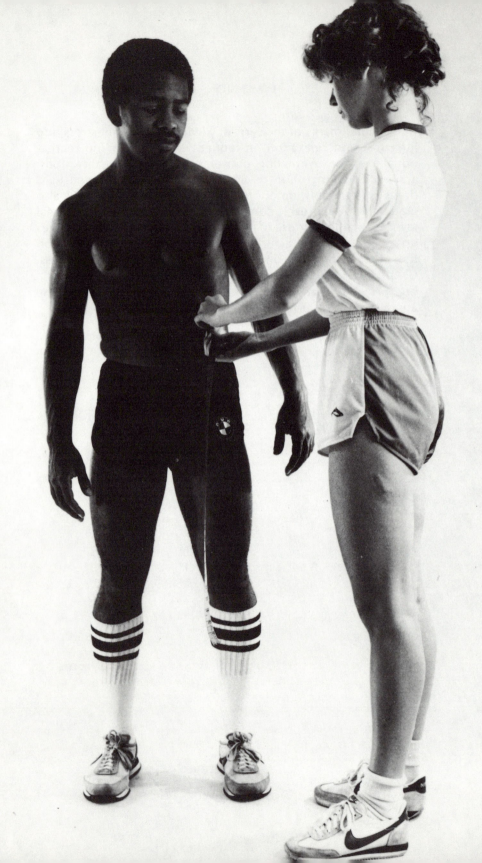

# Chapter Four

# PHYSICAL FITNESS APPRAISAL

*"That which is used develops, and that which is not used wastes away."*

*Hippocrates*

---

**KEY WORDS**

Fat Body Weight (FBW)      Overweight
Lean Body Weight (LBW)     Percent Body Fat (%BF)
Obesity                    Underweight

---

Each of us should know how physically fit he or she is. A general idea of one's fitness level can be gained most simply by reflecting on how well the body responds to the demands of the muscular work it performs periodically. Traditional (physiologic) measurements including body weight, waist circumference, resting heart rate, and blood pressure are also valuable fitness indicators. Such measures, in combination with the results of the basic fitness tasks that follow, will provide for an inclusive and objective appraisal of your state of physical fitness.

The practical techniques that have been selected to measure each component of fitness separately are neither time consuming nor intricate. They entail a minimum in the way of equipment and facilities; and many of them, once learned, can be repeated easily within and outside of the school environment. Additional fitness appraisals (including more scientific ones), although encouraged whenever possible, usually do require more elaborate procedures and sophisticated materials and facilities.

The physical fitness profile chart placed at the end of the chapter has been devised for the reporting and interpretation of your fitness data. When collected and recorded, the data should be scrutinized by your instructor. A comments section has been included for his or her written reactions and recommendations. Not only should fitness qualities in need of improvement be made clear to you, but the data should also prove useful in the determination of starting points (beginning dosage levels) in your physical activity regimens. Lastly, periodic fitness retesting is recommended (approximately every six to eight weeks) as a means of ascertaining fitness progress that might result from your exercise efforts.

# I. BODY LEANNESS EVALUATION

## A. COMPARISON OF BODY WEIGHT TO DESIRABLE WEIGHT

**Desirable (or Ideal) Weight** is an average body weight in pounds based on your sex, age, height, and body build. To be **overweight** simply means that you weigh more than your desirable weight. Obviously, **underweight** would imply your weighing less than the desirable weight. One should recognize at the outset that **obesity,** that is "excessive fatness," is not the same as overweight. The extra pounds that a lean, overweight person carries could very well be attributed to large, heavy bone and dense muscles (rather than to excessive body fat). On the other hand, many overweight people are indeed overfat;

and those who aren't have a strong tendency to become so later in life. Thus, the comparison of body weight to desirable weight is both a worthwhile and practical determination.

## Procedures

- Determine your height and weight in pounds (in shorts and T-shirt without shoes) using accurate instruments.
- Compare your body weight to the appropriate desirable weight in Tables 4.1 and 4.2, and determine if and by how many pounds you are overweight or underweight.
- Record the information in the Body Weight Measurement Chart.

### Table 4.1

### Desirable Weights for Men 20 to 30 Years Old (Weights Listed Without Clothing According To Height Without Shoes)*

| Height (feet, inches) | Weight (pounds) | | |
|---|---|---|---|
| | Low | Average | High |
| 5-3 | 123 | 129 | 135 |
| 5-4 | 127 | 133 | 139 |
| 5-5 | 131 | 137 | 143 |
| 5-6 | 136 | 142 | 148 |
| 5-7 | 140 | 147 | 154 |
| 5-8 | 144 | 151 | 158 |
| 5-8 | 149 | 155 | 162 |
| 5-10 | 153 | 159 | 166 |
| 5-11 | 156 | 163 | 171 |
| 6-0 | 160 | 167 | 175 |
| 6-1 | 164 | 171 | 180 |
| 6-2 | 168 | 175 | 184 |
| 6-3 | 171 | 178 | 188 |

*From U.S. Department of Agriculture: Food and your weight, Washington, D.C., 1973, U.S. Government Printing Office.

## Table 4.2

## Desirable Weights for Women 20 to 30 Years Old (Weights Listed Without Clothing According To Height Without Shoes)*

| Height (feet, inches) | Weight (pounds) | | |
|:---:|:---:|:---:|:---:|
| | Low | Average | High |
| 5-0 | 104 | 109 | 114 |
| 5-1 | 108 | 112 | 117 |
| 5-2 | 111 | 115 | 120 |
| 5-3 | 114 | 118 | 123 |
| 5-4 | 117 | 122 | 127 |
| 5-5 | 120 | 125 | 130 |
| 5-6 | 124 | 129 | 134 |
| 5-7 | 128 | 132 | 137 |
| 5-8 | 131 | 136 | 141 |
| 5-9 | 135 | 140 | 146 |
| 5-10 | 138 | 144 | 150 |
| 5-11 | 142 | 148 | 155 |
| 6-0 | 146 | 152 | 159 |

*From U.S. Department of Agriculture: Food and your weight, Washington, D.C., 1973, U.S. Government Printing Office.

## Body Weight Measurement Chart

| Date | Height (in.) | Body Weight (lbs.) | Desirable Weight (lbs.) | Lbs. Over- or Under- weight |
|---|---|---|---|---|
| | | | | |
| | | | | |
| | | | | |

# B. PERCENT BODY FAT (%BF) PREDICTION

### Criterion Measures and Standards

The percentage of total body weight that is fat (adipose) tissue, commonly called **Percent Body Fat,** is the best criterion measure for evaluating the quality of body weight. The most accurate methods of measuring %BF are hydrostatic weighing and water displacement. Both techniques involve submersion of the whole body within an expensive, specialized water container apparatus, which is unavailable to most of us. There- fore, several practical techniques (based on positive correla- tions with the more scientific ones) have been devised to estimate or predict percent body fat. One method of prediction incorporates the determination of circumferences (girths) of various body sites (such as the waist, forearm, thigh, buttocks, etc.) using a cloth tape measure. Such techniques, although quite practical, are not always accurate, especially among indi- viduals with muscular, athletic body builds. However, if class time permits and your instructor has access to requisite body site circumference formulas and tables*, by all means attempt to predict %BF via this method. If you do, compare your results to the techniques that follow. A portion of the physical fitness profile chart allots for the possibility of your completing body site circumference measurements.

One of the primary (structural-morphologic) differences between the sexes is that the female tends to be endowed with a greater amount of adipose tissue. Thus, common standards used to appraise states of body leanness in females are more stringent than for males. In a general sense, a condition of fatness exists for females with a body fat percentage **at or above 22 percent;** and for males **at or above 19 percent.**

Once the percentage of body fat is determined, **fat body weight (FBW)** and **lean body weight (LBW),** the actual pounds of fat and lean body tissues, can be easily calculated. The simple formulas are:

1. **FBW (lbs.)** $=$ %BF $\times$ Total Body Weight (lbs.)
2. **LBW (lbs.)** $=$ Total Body Weight (lbs.) $-$ FBW (lbs.)

---

*F. Katch and W. McArdle, *Nutrition, Weight Control, and Exercise* (Boston, Mass.: Houghton Mifflin Co., 1977), pp. 118-32.

Thus, a 160-pound person with 10 percent body fat has 16 pounds of body fat (FBW) and 144 pounds of lean body tissues (LBW) (10% of 160 = 16; and 160 − 16 = 144).

## 1. THE SIMPLE PINCH TEST

The most elementary indicator of percent body fat is the simple pinch test.

### Procedures

- Stand with exposed arms hanging in relaxed positions.
- Have a partner take a pinch of skin and underlying fat tissue (skinfold) in the center of the right upper arm halfway between the shoulder and the elbow. Make certain that none of the upper arm musculature is included in the skinfold.
- The pinch should be applied with the thumb and index finger of an inverted hand while measured (in inches) with a ruler held in the opposite hand (see photograph).

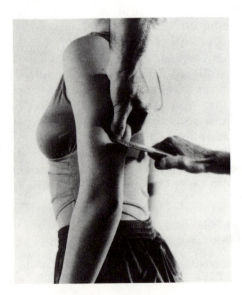

Simple pinch test

- Repeat the procedure with the left arm measured, and record the information in the Pinch Test Information Chart.
- Evaluate the average upper arm skinfold measurement as follows:

### Pinch Test Standards

| Sex | Upper Arm Skinfold Measurement | Indication |
|---|---|---|
| Male | > 6/8" | higher than normal %BF |
| Female | > 1" | |

### Pinch Test Information Chart

| Date | Upper Arm Skinfold (inches) Right   Left   Average | Higher Than Normal %BF Indicated (Yes or No) |
|---|---|---|
| | | |
| | | |
| | | |
| | | |

## 2. SKINFOLD THICKNESS MEASUREMENTS

This method of %BF prediction is the most preferable one. While it can be accomplished quickly, it does require the efforts of an instructor capable of taking the necessary thickness measurements with a skinfold caliper or other comparable device (as pictured).

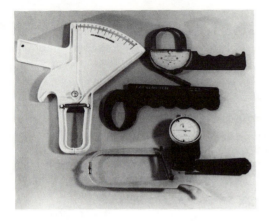

Instruments commonly used for skinfold thickness measurements

## Procedures

- Skinfold thickness measurements in millimeters (mm.) will be taken at three body sites for males **(Upper Arm, Chest,** and **Abdomen);** and two sites for females **(Upper Arm** and **Hip).** See the photographs provided for each.
- The tester should take two measurements at each site. A third one is to be taken only if the first two differ by more than three mm.

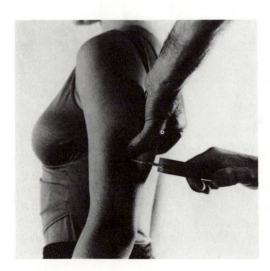

Upper arm skinfold: Back of the arm, halfway between the elbow and the top of the shoulder

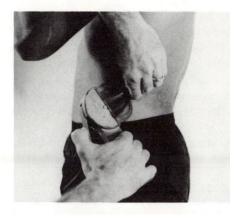

Hip skinfold: Side of the waist just above the pelvic bone

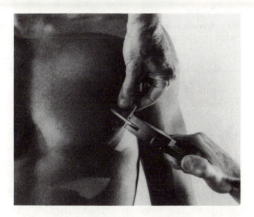

Chest skinfold: Just above and to the right of the nipple

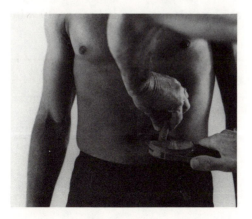

Abdomen skinfold: Just to the right of the navel

- The measurement is taken by pinching a full fold of skin and underlying fat tissue between the thumb and index finger of the inverted left hand. Caliper is held in the right hand. The fold should be held firmly and pulled away from deeper layers of muscle. Apply the caliper about a quarter of an inch below the fingers, which remain in position throughout the measurement. Read the dial after releasing the handles of the caliper.
- Record the data in the Skinfold Thickness Information Chart.

## Skinfold Thickness Information Chart

### Skinfold Thickness (mm.)

| Date | Female | | | Male | | | |
| | Upper Arm | Hip | Total | Upper Arm | Chest | Abdomen | Total |
|------|-----------|-----|-------|-----------|-------|---------|-------|
|      |           |     |       |           |       |         |       |
|      |           |     |       |           |       |         |       |
|      |           |     |       |           |       |         |       |

- Add the appropriate skinfold measurements and using the conversion chart (Table 4.3), estimate your percent body fat.
- Calculate your fat and lean body weight predictions (FBW and LBW) by following the formulas presented earlier in this chapter.
- Evaluate your body leanness using the Body Leanness Rating Chart.

## Body Leanness Rating Chart

| Leanness Rating | %BF Prediction | |
| | Male | Female |
|-----------------|------|--------|
| Excellent | 10 | 12 |
| Good | 11-15 | 13-20 |
| Fair | 16-19 | 21-23 |
| Poor | 20 | 23 |

● Record all body leanness information in the Body Leanness Information Chart.

### Body Leanness Information Chart

| Date | %BF Estimate | FBW (lbs.) | LBW (lbs.) | Body Leanness Rating |
|------|------|------|------|------|
|  |  |  |  |  |
|  |  |  |  |  |
|  |  |  |  |  |

# II. EVALUATION OF AEROBIC EFFICIENCY

## A. MEASUREMENT AND EVALUATION OF RESTING HEART RATE

In Chapter 2 we discussed that **heart rate (HR),** or **pulse rate** as it is also called, is the number of times the heart beats per minute. A low resting heart rate can, in a general sense, be indicative of a conditioned or fit heart and service network. Yet, it must also be realized that a high resting pulse rate does not necessarily imply low aerobic efficiency and a weak heart. One's heart rate at rest can be highly influenced by a variety of environmental and personal factors.

Although more detailed procedures for appraising aerobic efficiency do follow, let us begin our fitness appraisal by measuring heart rate accurately and evaluating our resting heart rate.

## Table 4.3

## Percentage Body Fat Conversion Chart*
### [Estimate from skinfolds (SF)]

| Female, total mm of SF [iliac (B) + triceps (A)] | Body Fat, % | Total SF, inches | Male, total mm of SF [mid ax. (C) juxt. nip. (D), triceps (A)] | Body Fat, % | Total SF, inches |
|---|---|---|---|---|---|
| 3.5 –   5.0 | 10 |      | 0.5 –   1.5 | 4 |      |
| 5.5 –   8.0 | 11 |      | 2.0 –   3.0 | 5 |      |
| 8.5 –  11.0 | 12 |      | 3.5 –   4.5 | 6 |      |
| 11.5 –  14.0 | 13 | ½″  | 5.0 –   6.5 | 7 | ¼″ |
| 4.5 –  17.0 | 14 |      | 7.0 –   8.5 | 8 |      |
| 17.5 –  19.5 | 15 |      | 9.0 –  12.0 | 9 |      |
| 20.0 –  22.5 | 16 |      | 13.5 –  17.5 | 10 |      |
| 23.0 –  25.5 | 17 | 1″  | 18.0 –  20.5 | 11 | ¾″ |
| 26.0 –  28.5 | 18 |      | 21.0 –  23.5 | 12 |      |
| 29.0 –  31.5 | 19 |      | 24.0 –  26.5 | 13 |      |
| 32.0 –  34.5 | 20 |      | 27.0 –  30.5 | 14 |      |
| 35.0 –  37.5 | 21 | 1½″ | 31.0 –  35.5 | 15 | 1½″ |
| 38.0 –  40.5 | 22 |      | 36.0 –  40.0 | 16 |      |
| 41.0 –  43.5 | 23 |      | 40.5 –  44.5 | 17 |      |
| 44.0 –  46.5 | 24 |      | 45.0 –  49.0 | 18 |      |
| 47.0 –  49.5 | 25 | 2″  | 49.5 –  53.5 | 19 | 2″ |
| 50.0 –  53.0 | 26 |      | 54.0 –  58.0 | 20 |      |
| 53.5 –  56.5 | 27 |      | 58.5 –  62.5 | 21 |      |
| 57.0 –  59.5 | 28 |      | 63.0 –  67.0 | 22 |      |
| 60.0 –  63.0 | 29 | 2½″ | 67.5 –  71.5 | 23 | 2¾″ |
| 63.5 –  66.5 | 30 |      | 72.0 –  76.0 | 24 |      |
| 67.0 –  69.5 | 31 |      | 76.5 –  80.5 | 25 |      |
| 70.0 –  73.0 | 32 |      | 81.0 –  85.0 | 26 |      |
| 73.5 –  76.5 | 33 | 3″  | 85.5 –  89.5 | 27 | 3½″ |
| 77.0 –  79.5 | 34 |      | 90.0 –  94.0 | 28 |      |
| 80.0 –  83.0 | 35 |      | 94.5 –  98.5 | 29 |      |
| 83.5 –  86.5 | 36 |      | 99.0 – 101.5 | 30 |      |
| 87.0 –  89.5 | 37 | 3½″ | 102.0 – 104.5 | 31 | 4¼″ |
| 90.0 –  92.5 | 38 |      | 105.0 – 107.5 | 32 |      |
| 93.0 –  95.5 | 39 |      | 108.5 – 112.0 | 33 |      |
| 96.0 –  98.5 | 40 |      | 112.5 – 116.5 | 34 |      |
| 99.0 – 101.5 | 41 | 4″  | 117.0 – 120.0 | 35 | 4¾″ |

*(continued)*

*Perry B. Johnson, et. al. *Sport, Exercise, and You* (New York: Holt, Rinehart, and Winston, 1975) pp. 6-64.

**Table 4.3** (continued)

| Female, total mm of SF [iliac (B) + triceps (A)] | Body Fat, % | Total SF, inches | Male, total mm of SF [mid ax. (C) juxt. nip. (D), triceps (A)] | Body Fat, % | Total SF, inches |
|---|---|---|---|---|---|
| 102.0 – 104.5 | 42 | | 121.5 – 125.5 | 36 | |
| 105.0 – 106.5 | 43 | | 126.0 – 130.0 | 37 | |
| 107.0 – 108.5 | 44 | | 130.5 – 134.5 | 38 | |
| 109.0 – 110.5 | 45 | 4½″ | 135.0 – 137.5 | 39 | 5½″ |
| 111.0 – 112.5 | 46 | | 138.0 – 141.5 | 40 | |
| 113.0 – 114.5 | 47 | | 142.0 – 143.5 | 41 | |
| 115.0 – 117.0 | 48 | | 144.0 – 148.0 | 42 | |
| 117.5 – 119.5 | 49 | 4¾″ | 148.5 – 152.5 | 43 | 6″ |
| 120.0 – 122.5 | 50 | | 153.0 – 157.0 | 44 | |
| | | | 157.5 – 161.5 | 45 | |
| | | | 162.0 – 166.0 | 46 | |
| | | | 166.5 – 170.5 | 47 | 6¾″ |
| | | | 171.0 – 175.0 | 48 | |
| | | | 175.5 – 179.5 | 49 | |
| | | | 180.0 – 185.0 | 50 | 7½″ |

## Procedures

- Assume a comfortable position (sitting quietly) for two to three minutes.
- Find your pulse by placing tips of index and middle fingers (either hand) on the carotid artery located on the side of the neck (just under the jaw and above the Adam's apple), or at the radial artery located at the thumb side of the wrist.
- Press in lightly and move the fingertips until the pulse is felt.
- Count the pulsations for fifteen seconds; then for thirty seconds; and then for one minute. Repeat pulse taking until the competency to take it is fully developed.
- Record the results on the Resting Heart Rate Information Chart, and evaluate your one-minute pulse rate using the Resting Heart Rate Rating Chart.

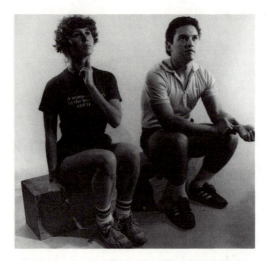

Students measuring heart rate: Neck (carotid) pulse, left; wrist (radial) pulse, right

## Resting Heart Rate Rating Chart

| Resting Heart Rate | Service Network Efficiency Rating (at rest) |
|:---:|:---:|
| 55 | Excellent |
| 56-65 | Very Good |
| 66-70 | Good |
| 71-80 | Average |
| 81-95 | Poor |
| 95 | Very Poor |

## Resting Heart Rate Information Chart

| Date | Method of Measuring Heart Rate | | | One Minute Resting Heart Rate Rating |
|---|---|---|---|---|
| | 15 Seconds | 30 Seconds | 1 Minute | |
| | | | | |
| | | | | |
| | | | | |

## B. AEROBIC EFFICIENCY EVALUATIONS BASED ON HEART RATE RESPONSE TO EXERCISE

Basically two kinds of field tests have been devised for the evaluation of aerobic efficiency. One category involves heart rate response to a specific exercise task. (Generally, the lower the heart rate elevation or the quicker its return to resting level, the more efficient the service network organs.) The second kind of test incorporates the ability to complete a demanding exercise or muscular work task at as high a rate of energy expenditure or work output as possible.

The performance of tests within the former category is more appropriate for all students in good health, because the exercise requirements are generally submaximal in both energy demands and stress to the service network. Thus, the two (HR response to exercise) tests that follow can be administered quite easily to varying groups of individuals, even prior to their commencing an aerobic physical activity conditioning program.

## 1. THE TWO-MINUTE, IN-PLACE JOGGING TEST

**Procedures**

- Take (and record) a thirty-second pulse rate after sitting quietly for two minutes.
- Jog in place for two minutes at a rate of three steps per second. A metronome set at 180 beats per minute will assure the proper jogging cadence (one step per beat). Raise each foot about three to five inches above the ground with every step.
- Immediately after the two-minute jogging period ends; sit and following 30 seconds take a 30 second heart rate.
- Inability to complete the two-minute jogging bout is a strong indication of very poor aerobic efficiency.
- Record the heart rate information and evaluate aerobic efficiency according to the Two-Minute, In-Place Jogging Test Rating Chart.

### Two-Minute, In-Place Jogging Test Rating Chart

| Difference in (30 Seconds) Resting and Post-Jogging Heart Rates | Aerobic Efficiency Rating |
|:---:|:---:|
| 0 | Superior |
| 1-3 | Excellent |
| 4-5 | Very Good |
| 6-7 | Good |
| 8-10 | Average |
| 11-15 | Poor |
| > 15 | Very Poor |

### Two-Minute, In-Place Jogging Test Information Chart

| Date | Post-Jogging 30-Second HR | Resting 30-Second HR | HR Difference | Aerobic Efficiency Rating |
|---|---|---|---|---|
|  |  |  |  |  |
|  |  |  |  |  |
|  |  |  |  |  |

## 2. THE STEP-UP TEST

**Procedures**

- Materials needed must be assembled. They include: a 12-inch step-up bench or platform, a clock or watch with a second-hand sweep, and a metronome (optional).
- Develop (by way of a practice session) the competency at the step-up maneuver described below.

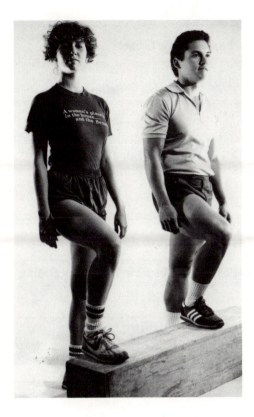

Students performing the step test

- Step up and down a 12-inch bench or platform at a rate of 24 steps per minute. A metronome, if available, can be set at 96 beats per minute (four beats per step) to help keep the proper stepping cadence. If unavailable, the tester can give verbal commands: "Up, up; down, down" (two steps per five seconds), to have the students maintain the correct stepping rate.
- Immediately following the three-minute step-up bout, the student sits down and quickly locates the pulse.
- A sixty-second heart rate is taken, starting no longer than five seconds after test completion. This recovery heart rate is your test score and is to be recorded in the Step-Up Test Information Chart.
- Recovery heart rate is to be evaluated in accordance to the Step-Up Test Rating Chart.

### Step-Up Test Rating Chart

| Age | | |
| Below 25 | Above 25 | Aerobic Efficiency Rating |
| --- | --- | --- |
| $< 75$ | $< 85$ | Excellent |
| 76-95 | 86-100 | Good |
| 96-105 | 101-115 | Fair |
| 106-110 | 116-125 | Poor |
| $> 110$ | $> 125$ | Very Poor |

### Step-Up Test Information Chart

| Date | Recovery HR Score | Aerobic Efficiency Rating |
| --- | --- | --- |
| | | |
| | | |
| | | |

## C. AEROBIC EFFICIENCY EVALUATION BASED ON PERFORMANCE OF A DEMANDING EXERCISE TASK: THE ONE AND ONE-HALF MILE RUN TEST

This is a timed test that requires your covering a distance of one and one-half miles (running, jogging, and/or walking) as quickly as possible. Since it involves a maximum effort with a high degree of stress placed on the heart and other service organs, it is an appropriate test for healthy persons who have been performing regular aerobic exercise for a minimum of five weeks. All others, especially those above age thirty, are cautioned in attempting this test. Only perform it when you are completely certain that you can handle its level of energy demands.

Any test participant who experiences extreme pain, dizziness, nausea, or weakness should discontinue the test immediately. No one should be forced to take the one and one-half mile run test against their will; and those participants who desire to discontinue it should be allowed to do so.

## Procedures*

- Warm up for a minimum of eight minutes.
- The total distance of one and one-half miles will involve six laps around a one-quarter mile track or seven and one-half laps around a one-fifth mile track. If neither track is available, a 100 or 200 yard square running course can easily be set up in almost any outdoor area. For the 100-yard square, the subject would complete 26 laps plus 40 yards; and for the 200-yard course, 13 laps plus 40 yards (in order to cover one and one-half miles).
- Students should work in pairs; one attempting the test and the other (standing in the start area) acting as a lap recorder. The instructor or other designated person) should act as the official timer, calling out the elapsed time periodically for all performers to hear.
- Following test completion, determine your aerobic efficiency rating (**Fitness Category**) based on the chart that follows.

## Aerobic Efficiency Rating Chart For The One and One-Half Mile Run Test

| Fitness Category | | Age (Years) | | | | | |
|---|---|---|---|---|---|---|---|
| | | 13-19 | 20-29 | 30-39 | 40-49 | 50-59 | 60 + |
| I. Very poor | (men) | > 15:31* | > 16:01 | > 16:31 | > 17:31 | > 19:01 | > 20:01 |
| | (women) | > 18:31 | > 19:01 | > 19:31 | > 20:01 | > 20:31 | > 21:01 |
| II. Poor | (men) | 12:11-15:30 | 14:01-16:00 | 14:44-16:30 | 15:36-17:30 | 17:01-19:00 | 19:01-20:00 |
| | (women) | 18:30-16:55 | 19:00-18:31 | 19:30-19:01 | 20:00-19:31 | 20:30-20:01 | 21:00-21:31 |
| III. Fair | (men) | 10:49-12:10 | 12:01-14:00 | 12:31-14:45 | 13:01-15:35 | 14:31-17:00 | 16:16-19:00 |
| | (women) | 16:54-14:31 | 18:30-15:55 | 19:00-16:31 | 19:30-17:31 | 20:00-19:01 | 20:30-19:31 |
| IV. Good | (men) | 9:41-10:48 | 10:46-12:00 | 11:01-12:30 | 11:31-13:00 | 12:31-14:30 | 14:00-16:15 |
| | (women) | 14:30-12:30 | 15:54-13:31 | 16:30-14:31 | 17:30-15:56 | 19:00-16:31 | 19:30-17:31 |
| V. Excellent | (men) | 8:37- 9:40 | 9:45-10:45 | 10:00-11:00 | 10:30-11:30 | 11:00-12:30 | 11:15-13:59 |
| | (women) | 12:29-11:50 | 13:30-12:30 | 14:30-13:00 | 15:55-13:45 | 16:30-14:30 | 17:30-16:30 |
| VI. Superior | (men) | < 8:37 | < 9:45 | < 10:00 | < 10:30 | < 11:00 | < 11:15 |
| | (women) | < 11:50 | < 12:30 | < 13:00 | < 13:45 | < 14:30 | < 16:30 |

*< Means "less than"; > means "more than."

*Kenneth Cooper, *The Aerobics Way* (New York: M. Evans and Co., 1977), p. 68 (Used with permission of the publisher).

Record results in the One and One-Half Mile Run Test Information Chart.

## One and One-Half Mile Run Test Information Chart

| Date | One and One-Half Mile Finishing Time | Aerobic Efficiency Rating (Fitness Category) |
|---|---|---|
| | | |
| | | |
| | | |

# III. EVALUATION OF LOCOMOTIVE NETWORK EFFICIENCY

Six basic pass-fail tests have been selected for the appraisal of this last component of physical fitness. The purpose and method of performance should be determined prior to attempting the completion of each test item.

## TEST ONE: THE PUSH-UP

**Purpose:** Measurement of minimal strength and stability of the upper arms, shoulders, and wrists.

**Procedures**

• Assume the front leaning rest position and hold for ten seconds. Maintain straight line from shoulders through hips, knees, and ankles.

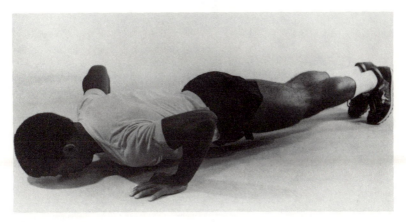

The push-up test

- Slowly lower the body in straight line by bending the elbows until only the nose contacts the ground.
- Hold this position for five seconds, and then slowly return to the starting position by extending the elbows, making sure to hold the straight body position.
- Inability to succeed in any phase of the task warrants failure.

**Result:** Check — Pass _____ Fail _____

## TEST TWO: TWO-HAND ANKLE GRAB

**Purpose:** Measurement of general body flexibility.

**Procedures**

- Assume standing position with heels together. Bend at the hips and knees slowly, bringing your arms between the knees and around the outside of the lower leg-ankle area.
- Continue until you reach a position of the hands being placed in front of the ankles with the finger tips interlocked.

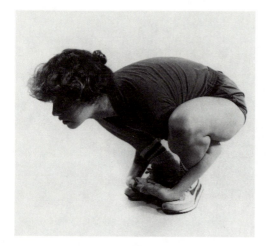

Two-hand ankle grab

- Maintain this position with interlocked finger tips for five seconds. The ability to attain and hold this position without falling over warrants a passing grade.

**Result:** Check — Pass _____ Fail _____

## TEST THREE: BENT-KNEE SIT-UPS

**Purpose:** Measurement of minimal strength and endurance of the abdominal musculature.*

### Procedures

- Lie on your back with the knees bent at a 90° angle, feet placed flat on the ground. Fold arms in front of the chest.

---

*The abdominal wall represents one of the most significant muscle groups within the body. Weakened abdominal muscles can result in a "sagging midsection" which is not only unattractive, but can easily precipitate an abnormal curvature of the back (lordosis), and the pain that accompanies it.

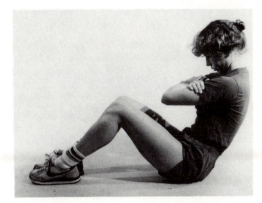

Bent-knee sit-up

- Maintaining this position, bring the torso up slowly so that the elbows touch the knees.
- Return slowly to the starting position.
- Complete 20 bent-knee sit-ups in a deliberate manner without bouncing. You must complete all 20 sit-ups to pass this test item.

**Result:** Check — Pass _____ Fail _____

# TEST FOUR: THE WALL TEST
# (LOW BACK PRESS)

**Purpose:** Determine lordosis, abnormal curve in the lower spine (sway-back).**

## Procedures

- Stand with the heels, backside, shoulders, and head contacting a straight wall.

---

**Failure implies possible lordosis which can easily lead to chronic low back pain. If such pain already exists, it would be wise to seek professional medical help. Corrective exercises might alleviate or prevent a compounding of the problem. Any physical activity that involves hyperextending the spine, that is, severe arching of the back, obviously could add to the abnormality, and should be avoided.

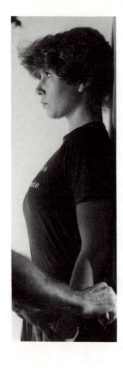

The wall test (low back press)

- Maintaining contact of these body areas with the wall, attempt to press the lower back flat against the wall.
- Have a partner attempt to gently slip (not force) a ruler between the lower back and the wall. If this can be done, you fail the test.

**Result:** Check — Pass _____ Fail _____

## TEST FIVE: DOUBLE DEEP KNEE BEND

**Purpose:** Measurement of minimal upper thigh strength, stability of the knee joint and leg bones.

**Procedures**

- Stand facing partner with feet about shoulder-width apart,

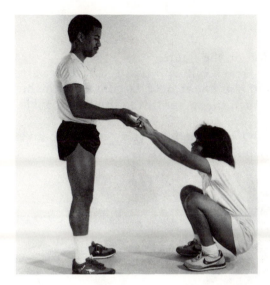

Double deep knee
bend

and pointing forward.
- Hold partner's hand (lightly for balance and support).
- Squat slowly, making sure to keep the back straight and the feet flat on the ground.
- Bend knees fully with the backside lowered to the heels. Hold this position for five seconds, maintaining a light grasp of your partner's hand for support balance only.
- Release partner's hand, and slowly raise up to starting position by extending the knees.
- Inability to perform any aspect of the test warrants failure.

**Result:** Check — Pass _____ Fail _____

## TEST SIX: SIT AND REACH

**Purpose:** Measurement of elasticity (capacity to stretch) of posterior thighs and flexibility of the spine and knees.*

---

*Excessive shortening of the posterior thigh muscles (hamstrings) can easily lead to tearing within these muscles when they are stretched. They tend to become shortened by remaining in the sitting position with the knees bent for long periods of time.

## Procedures

- Assume sitting position on the floor.
- Keeping the head up, reach out with outstretched, straight arms slowly, and with the knees held in contact with the ground, attempt to touch the finger tips to the inside ankle bones.
- Hold this position for five seconds. If you can do so, give yourself a passing grade.

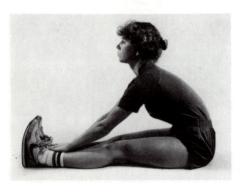

Sit and reach

**Result:** Check — Pass _____ Fail _____

- Rate your level of locomotive network efficiency according to the Locomotive Network Efficiency Rating Chart, and record all data in the Locomotive Network Efficiency Information Chart.

### Locomotive Network Efficiency Rating Chart

| Test Items Passed | Efficiency Rating |
|---|---|
| 6 | Excellent |
| 5 | Good |
| 4 | Fair |
| 3 | Poor |
| 2 or less | Very Poor |

## Locomotive Network Efficiency Information Chart

| Date | Number of Tests Passed | Locomotive Network Efficiency Rating |
|------|------------------------|--------------------------------------|
|      |                        |                                      |
|      |                        |                                      |
|      |                        |                                      |

# PHYSICAL FITNESS PROFILE CHART

## I. Personal Information

Last Name _____ First _____

Address _____

Phone _____ Age _____ Height _____

General Health Status _____

Known Health Problems (Disease, Handicap or Infirmity) _____

_____

## II. Body Composition and Leanness Information

### MEASUREMENT

| Date | Body Weight (lbs.) | Waist Circum-ference | Additional Circumference Measurements | | | % Body Fat Estimate |
|------|------|------|------|------|------|------|
| | | | 1._____ | 2._____ | 3._____ | (Circumference Measurement Technique) |
| | | | | | | |
| | | | | | | |

### MEASUREMENT

| Date | Skinfold Thickness Measurements | | | % Body Fat Estimate | %Body Fat Rating | LBW (lbs.) | FBW (lbs.) |
|------|------|------|------|------|------|------|------|
| | 1._____ | 2._____ | 3._____ | (Skinfold Thickness Technique) | | | |
| | | | | | | | |
| | | | | | | | |

## III. Aerobic Efficiency Information

### MEASUREMENT

| Date | Resting HR | Maximum HR | Blood Pressure** | | 2 Minute Jog Test Rating | Step Test Rating | One and One Half Mile Run | |
|------|-----------|-----------|-----------|-----------|----------|----------|----------|----------|
| | | | Systolic | Diastolic | | | Finishing Time | Rating |
| | | | | | | | | |
| | | | | | | | | |
| | | | | | | | | |

## IV. Locomotive Network Efficiency Information

### TEST ITEMS (Record pass or fail)

| Date | Push-up | 2-Hand Ankle Grab | Bent Knee Sit-ups | Wall Test | Double Knee Bend | Sit and Reach |
|------|---------|-------------------|-------------------|-----------|------------------|---------------|
| | | | | | | |
| | | | | | | |
| | | | | | | |

## V. Other Physical Fitness Tests

### TEST

| Date | 1. _____ | 2. _____ | 3. _____ | 4. _____ |
|------|-----------|-----------|-----------|-----------|
| | | | | |
| | | | | |
| | | | | |

## VI. Instructor Comments:

Date: _____

Date: _____

Date: _____

---

**If unable to have measured, check latest medical records.

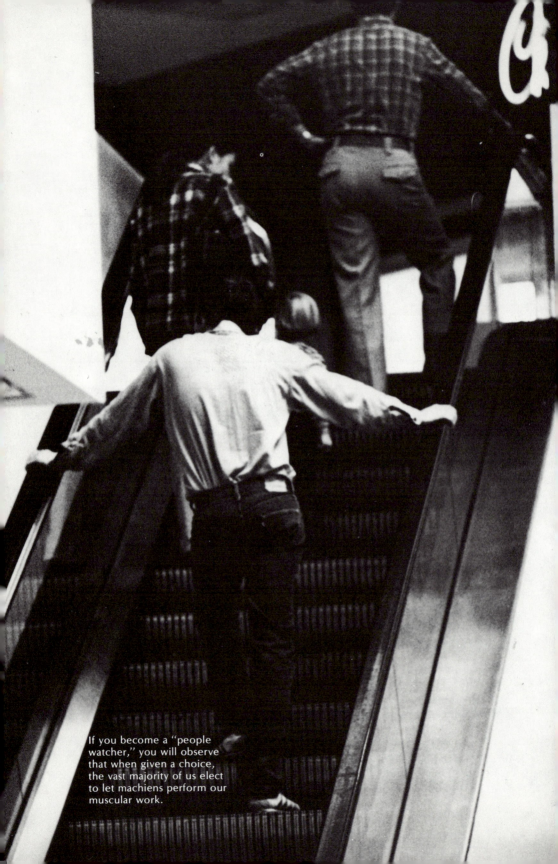

If you become a "people watcher," you will observe that when given a choice, the vast majority of us elect to let machiens perform our muscular work.

## Chapter Five

# PROPER EXERCISE: WHY AND HOW?

*"Most western nations are increasingly afflicted by a variety of pathological conditions, collectively designated as 'hypokinetic disease' which are attributable in a major or minor degree to the generally prevailing lack of exercise. These diseases, disorders, aches, and pains concern chiefly the muscular and cardiovascular systems, metabolism and emotional patterns."*

Hans Kraus and Wilhelm Raab

---

**KEY WORDS**

| | |
|---|---|
| Readiness | Balance |
| Specificity | Maintenance |
| Dosage | Work-out |
| Intensity | Warm-up |
| Duration | Cool-down |
| Frequency | Hyperventilation |
| Regularity | Side Stitch |
| Progression | Second Wind |
| Overload | Third Wind |

---

# REGULAR PHYSICAL ACTIVITY: IT CAN MAKE A DIFFERENCE

Let's backtrack a moment. It has been stated that exercise involves movements of the body (or body parts) through activation of the locomotive organs, mainly the skeletal muscles. When it is prolonged, the heightened muscle metabolism is sustained and controlled via operations within our service and regulatory networks. Your body should be taxed regularly with proper physical activity if it is to function more efficiently at rest and during periods of physical stress. In years past males and females of all ages were forced to exercise daily by carrying out many occupational and home-related duties. Technological advancement has just about put an end to that, especially among those of us who reside in large surburban and metropolitan areas. Now mechanical devices transport us from place to place, perform most of our demanding work tasks at home and on the job, and even provide us a variety of sedentary entertainment activities such as television viewing and radio listening. Thus, the total daily energy expenditure potential resulting from systematic activation of locomotive-service networks by way of either required or recreational physical activity has become quite low for much of our population.

Although the locomotive, service, and regulatory body organs proceed to grow and develop well into one's early adult years, they are composed of highly sensitive tissues. They will undoubtedly undergo structural, functional, and biochemical adaptations in response to both regular intervals of exercise and prolonged inactivity at every stage of life. Table 5.1 provides a comparison of the major physiological consequences that could result from the physically active and inactive life-styles.

# EXERCISE-RELATED DECISION MAKING

Each and everyone of you will make decisions and judgments relating to exercise at one time or another, beginning

## Table 5.1

## Potential Physiologic Adaptations Resulting From Regular Exercise and Prolonged Physical Inactivity

| | Potential Physiologic Adaptations | |
|---|---|---|
| **Body Organs and Tissues Affected** | **Prolonged Inactivity** | **Regular Exercise** |
| **Skeletal Muscles** | • Atrophy (shrinkage).<br>• Weakening and endurance reduction.<br>• Flabbiness and loss of tone or firmness (less supple musculature)<br>• Decreased elasticity<br>• Increased injury potential when stressed<br>• Weakening of abdominal musculature which leads to protrusion of visceral organs (sagging mid-section) which can precipitate sway back and backache. | • Strength-endurance development.<br>• Maintain or increase size muscle mass (Hypertrophy).<br>• Improved muscle firmness.<br>• Increased elasticity.<br>• Reduced risk of injury and orthopedic infirmity; especially heightened resistance to backache by maintaining above characteristics in back muscles which stabilize the spine; and abdominal muscles which better hold the visceral organs against the spine (less mid-section sagging). |
| **Bones and Joints** | • Lowered stability due to softening, weakening, and degeneration (osteoporosis); especially in those of middle age and beyond.<br>• Stiffness and flexibility reduction in major joints.<br>• Increased risk of sway back and back pain.<br>• Increased proneness to improper posture and body carriage.<br>• Increased proneness to injury and disability when stressed. | • Greater stability and stress resistance including that of spine.<br>• Promotes deposition of calcium within bones making them stronger and less vulnerable to degeneration and weakening. May delay or prevent osteoporosis.<br>• Leads to loose, flexible joints.<br>• Improved posture and body carriage.<br>• Greater resistance to orthopedic injury and disability.<br>• Stimulates bone marrow production of red blood cells.<br>• Improved circulation to bones, joints, and spinal disk preventing or delaying their deterioration. |

**Table 5.1** *(continued)*

| Potential Physiologic Adaptations | | |
|---|---|---|
| **Body Organs and Tissues Affected** | **Prolonged Inactivity** | **Regular Exercise** |
| Skin | • Decreased blood supply<br>• Loss of tissue density and elasticity. | • Increases flow of blood to skin to regulate internal body temperature during exercise.<br>• Greater potential for delivery of nutrients.<br>• Collagen content increases.<br>• Greater thickness, strength and elasticity.<br>• Fewer wrinkles, greater beauty, and healthy looking skin. |
| Service Network Organs (Heart, Lungs, Blood and Blood Vessels) | • Gradual weakening in muscular walls of the heart.<br>• Reduction in heart's blood pumping capacity at rest and during stress.<br>• Increased resting heart rate and increased heart rate response to exercise.<br>• Reduced blood flow to activated muscles.<br>• Reduced blood flow to heart walls during rest and exercise causing decreased metabolic functional efficiency of myocardium.<br>• Loss of elasticity in blood vessel walls.<br>• Lowered aerobic efficiency. | • Strengthens muscular walls of the heart.<br>• Increased heart pumping capacity at rest and during exercise.<br>• Decreased resting heart rate.<br>• Lowered heart rate response to exercise.<br>• Improved metabolic functioning of heart muscle - performs more work with less oxygen.<br>• Improved elasticity in walls of blood vessels.<br>• Increased maximum air intake capacity of lungs.<br>• Increased aerobic efficiency.<br>• Normalizes high blood pressure and can often decrease need to control it through medication.<br>• May increase blood volume. |
| **Internal and External Body Fat** | • Increase surface body fat (obesity).<br>• Promotes abdominal bulge or sagging mid-section and potential backache.<br>• Reduction in body's ability to dispose of harmful blood lipids (including cholesterol, triglyceride, and low and very low density lipoproteins). | • Decreased surface body fat (leanness).<br>• Reduces flab in mid-section and aids in the prevention of abdominal bulge, sway back and backache.<br>• Promotes body's ability to handle dangerous blood lipids.<br>• May help to prevent narrowing of critical blood vessels in heart and brain from build-up of fatty plaque on their walls. |

with the determination of whether to perform it or not. Unfortunately, far too many decide against exercising without weighing the significant information (such as the potential outcomes listed in Table 5.1). There are also great numbers among us who because of antiquated viewpoints and misinformation render decisions about exercise that defy logic. Some of you might insist that exercise is meant for highly fit or young people only, when in reality the benefits of proper physical activity can be reaped by all. And is it not the unfit individual leading a sedentary existence who has the most to gain by commencing a personalized physical fitness program? People who persist in the erroneous belief that it is either unfashionable or of insignificant value to exercise regularly should give their full consideration and reflection to the information reported in Table 5.1. All of you should also keep in mind that the dimensions of most of our physical attributes decline progressively after we reach our mid-twenties. You can either decelerate this decline through the systematic performance of proper exercise or accelerate it through sporadic or no exercise at all.

Let's also not neglect the fact that there are psychoemotional benefits of exercise which people of various cultures throughout the world have experienced since time immemorial. Suffice it to say that physical activity of every kind has always had an inherent human tranquilizing effect in that it can relieve tension, anxiety, and mental fatigue as well as providing participants needed fun and relaxation. **Thus, the potential of regular exercise in contributing to the fulfillment of human physiological, psychological, and sociological needs during these rather hectic, unsettling times makes it an essential ingredient of modern-day life.**

A word is warranted concerning those of you who do value fitness and exercise, but approach them unintelligently and unscientifically. Perhaps you are within that classification we might label as "weekend-athletes," who are most often ill-prepared for the stresses of physical activity sustained only on an occasional Saturday or Sunday. If so, it would be much wiser to condition your body for the rigors of weekend activities by several periods of weekday exercise. And lastly, we cannot fail to give consideration to the so-called "seekers of instant fitness!" That ever popular "get something for nothing" American philosophy has penetrated the confines of exercise and fitness and has led to the exploitation of a wide variety of wasteful, ineffective, and sometimes absurd commercial exercise-fitness enterprises. There are countless numbers of Americans who waste time and money on an ever-growing list of worthless, unnecessary, and often bizarre products and unproved schemes designed to strengthen muscles, firm up midsections, increase stamina, and remove unsightly fat without sweat, toil, or discomfort.

Typical Fitness Development Scheme

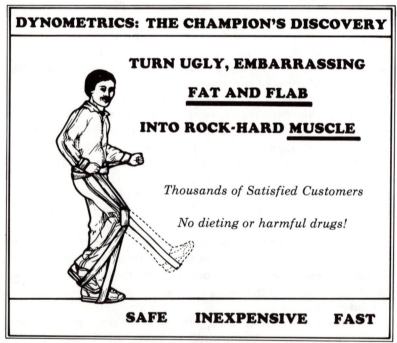

DYNOMETRICS: THE CHAMPION'S DISCOVERY

TURN UGLY, EMBARRASSING

FAT AND FLAB

INTO ROCK-HARD MUSCLE

*Thousands of Satisfied Customers*

*No dieting or harmful drugs!*

SAFE    INEXPENSIVE    FAST

Note:    Beware of fitness plans and products with miracle claims such as these.

**Figure 5.1**

In sum, it appears that too few of you can make intelligent judgments and effective choices concerning purposes, kinds, and amounts of exercise to perform. Let us begin to explore the information essential to avoid being mousetrapped by phony claims of exercise charlatans, and to develop the knowledge requisite to making sound decisions pertaining to fitness-related behaviors now and for the rest of your lives.

# ESSENTIALS OF PROPER EXERCISE

Proper exercise means safe, effective, and meaningful exercise that leads to the development and/or maintenance of optimal physical fitness with a minimum of problems or difficulties. It is more likely to be evidenced when one abides by the following guidelines and principles.*

## READINESS FOR EXERCISE

Every exerciser should be in a state of psychological and physiological readiness if benefits from physical activity are to be realized. Common sense dictates that the kinds and amount of physical activity to perform be in line with your unique nature including the capacity to handle the stress of the exercise selected. In holding to this relevant principle, if you are under thirty years of age without symptoms of disease or disability, and free from medical limitations as of your last examination by a physician, you can commence a suitable exercise program with few restrictions. On the other hand, a medical checkup prior to embarking in exercise would be appropriate if there might be some doubt about your health status. Examination by a physician becomes a more significant prerequisite to exercise for those of you above age thirty — especially if you have been leading a sedentary life.

Certain forms of exercise are not always appropriate for some people. In cases where physical shortcomings are known to exist (or are revealed through a medical exam), the rigors of physical activity could possibly cause more harm than good. Those with a serious heart ailment, for example, might be restricted completely from participating in exercise of any form. Physically handicapped persons are often limited in terms of what types of movement they are capable of performing. Victims of backache attributed to weakened (abdominal and

---

*A principle is simply a piece of factual or accepted information used to direct behavior.

back) muscles and tight joints in the spine very often respond positively to specified exercise tasks for their condition. But others whose back pain is caused by a ruptured vertebral disk, could very well aggravate their problem by adherence to the very same exercise routine. In short, when it seems warranted, seek the advice and direction of a medical authority who can only help you make proper decisions relating to a suitable personal exercise prescription.

In addition to physiological readiness, the person about to commence an exercise program should be motivated to do so; that is he or she recognizes the need and intrinsic worth of proper physical activity (psychological readiness).

## THE SPECIFICITY PRINCIPLE

Any physiological adaptation resulting from exercise (see Table 5.1) tends to be related exclusively to the particular organs and tissues stressed by the exercise task. The degree of change produced is also dictated to some degree by the extent to which these areas are affected by exercise. For example, aerobic efficiency will be improved by the performance of aerobic physical activities, while anaerobic ones will develop anaerobic energy producing mechanisms, The development of flexibility within a joint necessitates short bouts of progressive tendon, ligament, and muscle stretching. (This relevant principle will be reiterated in subsequent chapters since it provides the basis for the classification of exercise-fitness programs.)

## REGULARITY AND PROGRESSION

**Regularity** and **progression** are common sense, yet frequently neglected principles. To better comprehend their meaning we must introduce the concept of exercise dosage, a word used to quantify exercise. **Dosage, the amount of exercise performed in one week,** is a composite of three major variables as depicted below.

## Exercise Dosage

How much exercise
performed in one week

| INTENSITY | DURATION | FREQUENCY |
|---|---|---|
| Metabolic demands, requirements or stress of exercise performed. | Time involved in an exercise period or work-out. | Number of exercise periods or work-outs per week. |

Intensity reflects the degree of physical stress or metabolic demands created by a particular exercise task. It involves your body's physiological responses to the movement patterns being performed. Energy expenditure (kilocalories per minute or hour) and heart rate, an indication of the degree of service network activation, are the most common criteria utilized in measuring exercise intensity. In fact, heart rate is a very practical and useful tool for setting and adjusting intensity, since it is a physiological measurement you can attain with little difficulty. However, certain fitness authorities feel that your psychological

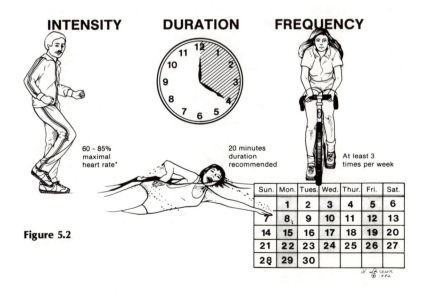

**INTENSITY**  
60 - 85% maximal heart rate*

**DURATION**  
20 minutes duration recommended

**FREQUENCY**  
At least 3 times per week

**Figure 5.2**

| Sun. | Mon. | Tues. | Wed. | Thur. | Fri. | Sat. |
|---|---|---|---|---|---|---|
|  | 1 | 2 | 3 | 4 | 5 | 6 |
| 7 | 8 | 9 | 10 | 11 | 12 | 13 |
| 14 | 15 | 16 | 17 | 18 | 19 | 20 |
| 21 | 22 | 23 | 24 | 25 | 26 | 27 |
| 28 | 29 | 30 |  |  |  |  |

feelings and perception of the relative degree of exertion experienced during exercise are a more individualized and safe exercise intensity indicator* (Table 5.2). This will be discussed in greater detail in Chapter 10. Duration represents the time utilized in one exercise period. The number of periods performed per week is signified by the work "frequency."

If the human need for exercise is as vital as that of sound nutrition, then exercise, like eating, should be performed with regularity rather than sporadically. Although the dosage and

---

*Phillip Hage, "Perceived Exertion: One Measure of Exercise Intensity," *The Physician and Sports Medicine* (McGraw-Hill Publication), September 1981, pp. 136-46.

## Table 5.2

## Typical Criteria for the Classification of Exercise Intensity

| Exercise Intensity Classification | Criteria Heartrate | Energy Expenditure (Kcal./hour) | Perceived Exertion |
|---|---|---|---|
| Very light | < 110 | < 110 | very, very easy |
| Light | 110 - 120 | 111 - 270 | easy, no pain discomfort |
| Moderate | 121 - 150 | 270 - 400 | somewhat difficult and slight discomfort |
| Heavy | 151 - 160 | 401 - 550 | difficult, discomfortable and some pain |
| Very heavy | 161 - 180 | 550 - 699 | very difficult and painful |
| Exhaustive | > 180 | > 700 | extreme difficulty and pain |

mode of physical activity may vary, it is this author's contention that each one of you should eventually reach a state of readiness that allows you to perform some form of recreational exercise on a daily basis. By no means is this meant to imply, however, that you must exercise to your maximum capacity each and every day. But if on a particular day you have time for only a fifteen-minute walk or jog, you should not pass up this opportunity. Exercise selection, a topic that is discussed more fully in Chapter 10, depends on a host of factors in addition to time availability.

Progression simply means that the initial dosage when commencing a fitness program be geared to your state of physiological readiness, without threat to health or body impairment. Then as your level of physical fitness improves, dosage variables could be gradually elevated. A safe starting point depends mainly on your health, age, and previous exercise patterns. For example, sedentary people might best begin with ten-minute bouts of very light to light intensity physical activity performed every other day. And regardless of your fitness condition and degree of advancement in any exercise program, it is an intelligent and sensible precaution to do too little rather than too much exercise on any one occasion. Upgrading of functional capacities within your service and locomotive networks will eventually occur in response to gradually heightened requirements made of them via progressive dosage increases. However, you should take the time to elevate exercise demands slowly, because too much exercise too soon could produce a number of different debilitating conditions. As a matter of fact, overdoing it (overstress) at any stage of fitness development is often the major culprit in the onset of chronic tiredness and fatigue; lowered resistance to germs; local muscle-joint soreness, stiffness, and inflammation; and even stress fractures of bones (Chapter 9). But it must also be recognized that few if any permanent physiological benefits are derived from sporadic or infrequent exercise.

## THE OVERLOAD PRINCIPLE

The **overload principle,** perhaps, may be the most difficult exercise concept for you to understand theoretically and to apply in practice. The following series of events should foster your comprehension of it. An exercise routine involving jogging at five miles per hour for twenty minutes, four times weekly, caused a gradual reduction in the performer's exercise heart rate from 150 to 135. After six weeks of this regimen, subsequent heart rate decrements failed to occur. The performer then elevated the intensity and duration of the exercise program by jogging at seven miles per hour for thirty minutes, four times weekly. Following several weeks of conditioning with this dosage, the original jogging task (at previous intensity of 5 mph) was again attempted. This time, however, a decline in exercise heart rate to 130 was experienced by the jogger. The implication here is that the heightened exercise dosage (jogging at a faster rate) was responsible for the production of service network adaptations reflected in the decreased heart rate that took place. We commonly refer to this progressive upgrading of total metabolic requirements of exercise (via dosage increments) as progressive overload. Keep in mind that for every form of exercise task, overload is a primary requisite to the improvement of the specific fitness mechanisms you are utilizing.

Overload can result from the elevation of one or more of the three dosage variables. Intensity increments represent the most stressful application of overload, and are most suited to individuals of average and above average fitness levels. It is more appropriate for any person with a fitness status that falls below the fair to moderate degree (especially the elderly and/or sedentary) to increase exercise dosage by way of duration and frequency elevations.

Warranting discussion at this point is the fact that the relationship between degree of overload and physiological response produced is not linear. Some of you may mistakenly think that by doubling or tripling your exercise dosage, you will double or triple the gains derived in physical fitness. For example, let's say that the adherence to an aerobic exercise program (involving twenty minutes of jogging at five miles per hour completed three times weekly) produces a five percent improvement in your service network efficiency as indicated by a specific aerobic efficiency test. Jogging at ten miles per hour for forty minutes, six times per week over the same course of time would not necessarily produce a ten percent increase in service network efficiency.

There is a great deal of variation from individual to individual in the rate and magnitude of physiological adaptation within fitness organs resulting from overload conditioning. Obviously, the poorer your original state of physical fitness prior to regular exercise, the greater the potential for its improvement. Remember that if you have been previously inactive, your very first attempt at exercise is in reality one of overload. Although it is an essential requirement for the production of improvements in major fitness mechanisms, when excessive, overload can cause harmful and debilitating effects to your body.

## FITNESS BALANCE AND MAINTENANCE

The balance principle implies that each component of physical fitness be optimally developed through an effective, well-rounded exercise program. A balanced exercise regimen is one that incorporates physical activities designed to enhance aerobic efficiency as well as flexibility and strength-endurance levels of the major muscle-joint areas of the body. (Fortunately, all forms of exercise promote body leanness in that they heighten energy production; but more about this in Chapter 8.)

The term balance in the context of fitness also connotes the idea that the strength-endurance capacities of opposition muscle groups (that is those involved in movement of limbs in opposite directions) within the critical joints of the body be equal. Constant repetition of the same movement patterns from participation in the same physical activity can often lead to the overdevelopment of the muscles and joints activated, and the underdevelopment of other local muscle-joint areas not utilized. Eventually the activated tissues grow stronger and begin to dominate the neglected, weaker ones. Walking, jogging, and running, for example, tend to overdevelop the musculature of the anterior thigh and the lower posterior leg or calf muscles while providing little activation for the posterior thigh and anterior portion of the lower legs. Naturally these weaker muscles become prone to strain. A muscle strain, commonly called a "pulled muscle," involves a rupturing or tearing of muscle tissue that can be quite painful and incapacitating. Actually this may be why portions of the group of three muscles that constitute the posterior thigh, the "hamstrings," are so frequently strained while jogging or running. The "hamstrings" serve to control and brake knee extension, which is produced in running activities via the contraction of the anterior thigh musculature, the "quadriceps." This group of four muscles composing the anterior thigh, the most powerful group within the body, can contract with such a degree of violent tension that the less powerful tissues of the "hamstrings" are actually torn in their attempts to brake the forceful knee extension being produced.

A highly specialized exercise prescription might be warranted when you recognize a severe fitness weakness. However, if major deficiencies do not exist or if there is room for improvement in all your fitness attributes, a balanced exercise program should be designed. The term maintenance indicates that when fitness proceeds to your desired level, progressive overload can ease with exercise dosage remaining fairly constant. Those of you who achieve a state of fitness that you can maintain through daily exercise will find it highly rewarding psychologically and physically.

# "WORKING-OUT"

There are actually three distinct phases of an exercise bout, or "work-out" as it is more commonly called. They include the **warm-up, body, and cool-down. The longest portion during which the most intense demands are generated among loco-motive and service organs is the body of the work-out.** Regardless of the mode of exercise you are going to perform, it is wise to precede the body of the work-out with a solid eight to fifteen minute warm-up period. This is time that is well-spent in that it will better prepare you both physiologically and psychologically for the more stressful action that will follow. Athletes and dancers have long recognized the values of warming-up in terms of both performance and safety (injury prevention). Many of the internal physiological adjustments to the exercise state, although automatic, require a few minutes to be fully set into operation. Basic warm-up tasks, which include walking, slow jogging, and calisthenics (jumping jacks, trunk bending, half-squats, etc.), will elevate your core (internal) temperature by activating your large skeletal muscles while setting service and regulatory mechanisms into motion. The gradual acceleration in heart rate that results is an indication that a heightened volume of blood has begun to be pumped from your heart. Blood vessels within the lungs and working muscles and joints will start to widen automatically (via regulatory messages from brain centers) to receive the increased blood flow, thus magnifying the passage of nutrients and wastes between activated tissues and blood vessels. Heat generated within soft tissues (of muscles and joints) reduces their viscosity (thickness) and resistance to movement. Thus, seven minutes or so into the warm-up period, you can safely begin to devote efforts toward progressive stretching tasks including heel cord, hamstring, and quadriceps stretches (see pages 139-140).

Impulse messages within your brain and spinal cord will travel with greater frequency and speed and will be relayed to one another more readily as higher core temperatures are initiated. Hence, there is an elevated level of (neuromotor) control of movement patterns which should be evidenced by your improved skill capacity. And lastly, to use some modern-day jargon, after warm-up you are more likely to be "psyched-up" for the strenuous exercise to occur during the body of your work-out.

Another period of about ten minutes or more following more intense exercise, called cool-down, should be utilized for gradual heat dissipation and more extensive muscle-joint stretching. The continuation of light intensity exercise tasks (walking, slow jogging, calisthenics) at this time sustains the circulation of heated blood to your skin cooling centers which in turn promotes your body's return to a normal internal temperature level. Stretching muscles and joints facilitates their recovery and counters tightness and soreness precipitated within them from the constant production of the same ballistic movement patterns. Please note that cool-down stretching tasks should be more intense, longer in duration, and more inclusive in number than your warm-up stretches. Since the elevated body temperature and muscle-joint usage tend to promote the elasticity of soft locomotive tissues, the potential for increasing both your range of joint motion and muscle lengthening is the greatest toward the end rather than at the beginning of an exercise work-out.

# POTENTIAL NEGATIVE AND POSITIVE SENSATIONS EXPERIENCED DURING EXERCISE

## HYPERVENTILATION AND "SECOND-WIND"

Over the years, many students have raised the question of how they should breathe during sustained exercise activities such as jogging. Respiration happens to be one of the more automatically controlled physiological responses of your body (Autonomic Nervous System). In actuality, breathing adjustments during exercise if left alone should occur on their own. What definitely is to be avoided is any attempt at rapid, deep breathing *(hyperventilation)* which many of you force yourselves to do both before and during exercise. Such efforts heighten the energy requirements of the muscles associated with the production of breathing, and are thereby draining to your body's overall energy reserve.

You might have noticed that some degree of involuntary hyperventilation seems to be experienced during the first minutes of exercise, producing feelings that range from mild discomfort to extreme pain (dyspnea). These rather negative feelings are especially disheartening to the unfit person who after long periods of neglect commences an exercise program. Fact is that poorly conditioned individuals become "winded" more readily and remain that way for a longer period of time than fit people.

Generally with the continuation of exercise, breathing, although elevated, becomes more rhythmic and less burdensome. The occurrence of this natural respiratory phenomenon called **second wind** not only involves the dissipation of feelings of discomfort, but often generates a renewed capacity and desire to continue exercise. There are no magical styles or

Common Sensations Experienced during Exercise

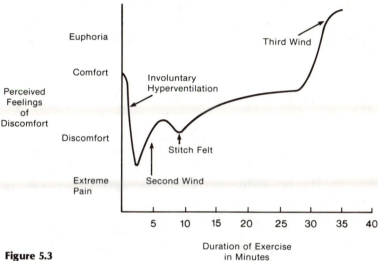

**Figure 5.3**

techniques of breathing that will eliminate the breathing difficulties that you might experience during the early stages of
sustained exercise. The response may take a few minutes to
occur, but with a little patience and perseverance the unfit
beginner like the exercise veteran will experience the miracle
of second wind. And observation indicates that with the passage
of time, as physical fitness improves through systematic exercise, any breathing difficulties should subside.

## CONCENTRATION ON BREATHING DURING EXERCISE

While discussing respiration, one last significant point warrants mention. Many seasoned exercisers have found that
concentration on breathing is quite helpful to their performance of a variety of physical activities. Focusing on slow,
steady inhalation and exhalation of air that are occurring
naturally while performing sports, jogging, swimming, stretch-

ing, and calisthenic routines, tends to divert the mind's attention from both distractions and uncomfortable feelings. Thus, the overall performance of the physical activity is enhanced along with one's psychological perception of it. Concentrating on your breathing patterns in your next work-out may be worth a try!

## SPEED STARTS AND PACING

At any stage of a work-out, if the intensity level of exercise becomes excessive, oxygen and fuel will not be supplied to highly activated muscles quickly enough to meet their energy demands. This results in waste buildup and associated negative feelings which tend to be quite incapacitating. When commencing any exercise task that you intend to sustain for a long period of time (such as a distance run, swim, or bicycle ride), quick, speedy starts are to be avoided. Far better to pace yourself; that is to start with more moderate speeds which could be maintained for a long duration of time, and increase intensity gradually at the middle and latter stages of the work-out when the body is fully warmed-up and ready for handling greater demands for energy production.

## "THE SIDE-STITCH"

Another unpleasant sensation not uncommon to exercisers during their initial work-outs is the **"side-stitch," that stabbing pain felt on your side near the bottom of the rib cage.** Sometimes it can become so excruciating, it will force you to either cease activity completely or to slow the pace considerably. Speculation is that the stitch is actually a spasm within your diaphragm muscle that could be attributed to any number of reasons ranging from prolonged heavy breathing to the muscle's extreme sensitivity to a lack of oxygen. Improving physical fitness through regular exercise, proper warm-up, pacing yourself, and avoidance of heavy eating and/or drinking prior to exercise, promotes second wind, reduces the chances of developing a side-stitch, and assures a more positive overall exercise experience.

# THE "EXERCISE HIGH" AND
# PHYSICAL ACTIVITY ADDICTION

A more positive sensation experienced often by long distance runners, cyclists, and swimmers some twenty-five minutes or more into their work-out is the phenomenon of **"third wind." Basically it is a feeling of euphoria (well-being) and renewed confidence in one's capacity to meet the demands of the exercise task being performed.** Conjecture is that third wind, more recently referred to as the "exercise high," is due mainly to a series of internal biochemical events that occur automatically during sustained exercise efforts. Glucose, it might be recalled, is the primary fuel utilized by muscles during the initial stages of exercise. However, with sustained physical activity the energy for muscle contraction is provided by the oxidation of fat (in the form of free fatty acids). The conversion of fat to its usable form and its transfer from fat tissues to muscle cells via the blood requires time. The third wind sensation in part might be attributed to the utilization of fat as the sole source of energy for muscle contraction.

More recently there has been a great deal of discussion relating to the release of hormones called beta-endorphins within the brain during periods of sustained exercise. Authorities theorize that these biochemical substances might somehow produce positive psychological feelings or an "exercise high," and that they may be addictive. People who engage in sustained physical activity with great frequency may do so in part because their bodies crave the release of these mood-elevating hormones. When exercise is curtailed for one reason or another, there is a strong tendency for a depressed, unhappy state of mind to result which could be attributed to the brain's failure to produce beta-endorphins.

**Regardless of causation, the fact remains that more and more people seem to be experiencing a psychological "high" through the frequent performance of long duration exercise. And if exercise is indeed addictive, wouldn't you be fortunate to become compelled to do something which is physiologically beneficial, rather than to be addicted to the likes of excessive food, gambling, cigarettes, alcohol, or hard drugs?**

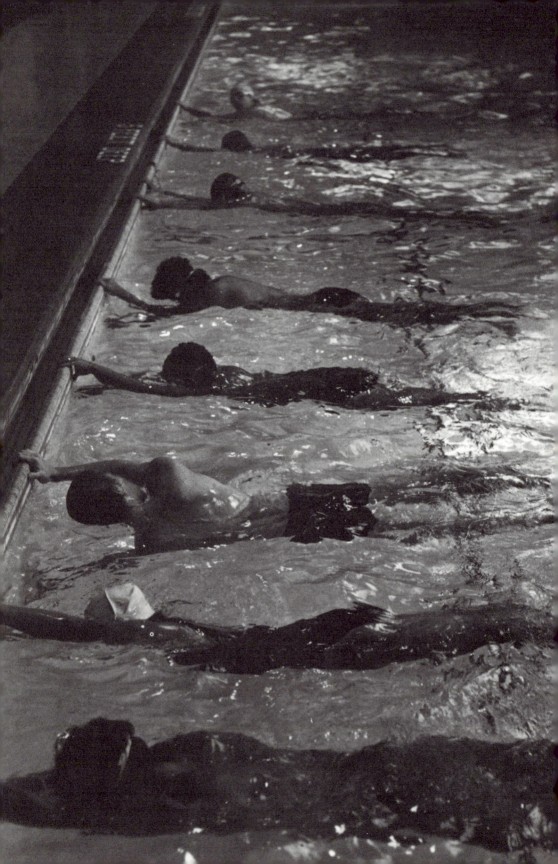

# Chapter Six

# AEROBIC PHYSICAL ACTIVITY PROGRAMS

*"Reading is to the mind,*
*what exercise is to the body."*

*Richard Steele*

---

**KEY WORDS**

Aerobic Endurance

Aerobic Power

Maximum Heart Rate ($HR_{max}$)

Critical Threshold (CT)

Target Heart Rate.(THR)

Continuous Exercise

Internal Conditioning

---

## THE CONSIDERATION OF POPULAR MODES OF PHYSICAL ACTIVITY

There are literally hundreds of different ways to exercise your body, ranging from traditional conditioning tasks to the performance of household chores. You can do so in standing, sitting, and lying positions — on land, in water, or over ice and snow. Highly specialized facilities, equipment, and movement skills are necessary for many popular physical activities (such as downhill skiing and swimming). For the more elementary, uncomplicated ones (none more simple than walking), few requirements exist. As a matter of fact, if you desired to do it, you could easily carry out a meaningful physical fitness program without any special equipment or clothing, within the confines of your living room.

In terms of exercise regimens, some people prefer to follow more rigid, structured plans devised by fitness experts, while others of us choose to construct programs of our own. It would be impossible to detail within this text every possibility for exercise that exists. However, essential positive and negative features of the more popular modes of physical activity (discussed in this chapter and the following one) are indeed warranted. Such information will enhance an intelligent selection of physical activity for your own personalized fitness development.

Before proceeding further, let me reemphasize that a **well-rounded program of exercise (balance principle), regardless of the means by which it is accomplished, should include provision for the development or maintenance of: (1) aerobic efficiency; (2) strength, endurance, and flexibility of major locomotive areas of the body; and (3) body leanness.** Remember, these aspects of physical fitness are highly interrelated! Thus, while a certain type of physical activity program generally develops a particular fitness characteristic (principle of specificity), it will affect others as well — sometimes extensively and at other times minutely. Ballet is a classic example of a mode of exercise that

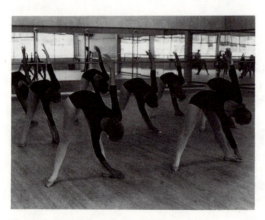

**Table 6.1**

**Reminders for All Exercisers**

- Always exercise at a dosage level your body can tolerate.
- Get into your exercise program gradually. Better to do too little than too much physical activity during a workout.
- Progress with dosage increments in line with your fitness needs, goals, and physiological readiness.
- Strive for balance in fitness development.
- Warm up adequately before submitting your body to more stressful movements and energy demands.
- Cool down and stretch out following more extensive activity.

can concurrently foster muscle strength-endurance levels, joint flexibility, and aerobic efficiency. Finally, regardless of the type of physical activity you perform, let your efforts and actions be in line with guidelines previously discussed in Chapter 5 and summarized in Table 6.1.

# FEATURES OF AEROBIC EXERCISE

Aerobic efficiency, as explained earlier, is the service network's capacity to supply fuel and oxygen-enriched blood continuously to activated locomotive organs during exercise. Muscles of the body can better sustain periods of elevated energy demand when they receive an adequate supply of blood. Conversely, if the volume of blood delivered to activated locomotive tissues is negligible, energy production within them falters, and the capacity to endure the exercise task becomes limited.

While it is the nature of all aerobic physical activities to elevate heart rate for a substantial period of time, they can range quite widely from low- to high-power types. **Lower power, or aerobic endurance development exercise,** obviously elevates heart rate minimally. It is designed mainly to enhance the participant's ability to sustain lower energy demands created by lighter intensity physical activity. Upgrading exercise dosage for the sole purpose of improving your aerobic endurance is best accomplished via progressive increments in duration and/or frequency variables rather than through intensity.

**Evidently, aerobic power activities are more strenuous in nature and thus heighten service network activation well beyond the level of typical aerobic endurance activities.** In fact, in order to be intense enough to cause functional improvements within power mechanisms of the service network, they must cause the exercise heart rate to climb to a minimal target level. This minimal exercise heart rate, commonly referred to as **critical threshold, is believed to be 70 percent of the exerciser's maximum heart rate. Maximum heart rate (HR$_{max}$), the highest number of times the heart can beat per minute,** can be estimated quite easily by subtracting your age in years from the

## Table 6.2

## Guidelines for Construction of Aerobic Endurance and Power Exercise Programs

| Program Classification | Outcome | Intensity | Duration | Frequency |
|---|---|---|---|---|
| Aerobic Endurance | 1. Maximum improvement in the capacity to sustain exercise of light intensity levels.<br><br>2. Minimum improvement in aerobic power. | Very light to light: Physical activities selected must *not* be too strenuous but must be light enough in energy demand to be sustained for the duration of each workout. | 1. Initial workouts should range between 8-20 minutes.<br><br>2. Progressive lengthening until capable of sustaining workout of desired pre-set level (e.g., 30-60 min.). | 1. Initial workouts performed minimum of 3 times/week.<br><br>2. Progressive increments until pre-set goal is reached (e.g., 5-7 times per week). |
| Aerobic Power | 1. Improvement in aerobic power.<br><br>2. Improvement in the capacity to sustain high intensity exercise. | Intense enough to cause heart rate elevation to 70-90% of maximal heart rate. | 1. Initial workouts of 10 min. or more.<br><br>2. Progressive lengthening until pre-set goal reached (e.g., 30-60 min.). | 1. Initial workouts performed 3 times/week.<br><br>2. Progressive increments until pre-set goal accomplished (e.g., 4-5/week). |

number 220.* In actuality, one's target heart rate (THR) during the performance of aerobic power exercise can range from 70-90 percent of $HR_{max}$. It could be appropriately selected in light of your present level of aerobic fitness as follows:

| Aerobic Fitness Level | % $HR_{max}$ |
|:---:|:---:|
| Low | 70 |
| Moderate | 71-80 |
| Excellent | 81-90 |

Thus, in designing an aerobic power exercise program, a moderately fit twenty-year-old would determine the THR as follows:

**Formula: THR** = 80% $HR_{max}$    .80 × 200 = 160.

Basic guidelines for program construction of both categories of aerobic exercise appear in Table 6.2.

# CONTINUOUS AND INTERVAL AEROBIC EXERCISE PROGRAMS

Aerobic physical activities can be performed in either a constant or **"steady state" with little fluctuation in energy output or intermittently, that is, with alternating periods of high and low energy demands.** In the steady state method, which is also termed **continuous exercise,** your heart rate would be made to rise to a particular level but would then remain relatively close to it throughout the duration of the work-out. The reverse, however, is true for intermittent exercise, more popularly known as **interval conditioning.** Here, heart rate, in responding to the alternating levels of energy demand, assumes

---

*Age is subtracted from this recommended number because your maximum heart rate decreases progressively with age. The simple formula is $HR_{max} = 220 -$ age. Thus, the $HR_{max}$ for a 20-year old is 200; for a person of age 40, it is 180.

Comparison of Heart Rates Attained in Continuous
and Interval Exercise for Aerobic Endurance and Power

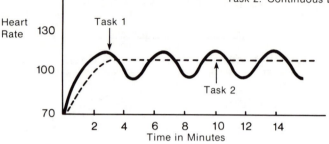

A. AEROBIC ENDURANCE DEVELOPMENT: Task 1: Interval Exercise
Task 2: Continuous Exercise

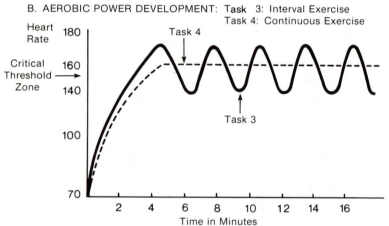

B. AEROBIC POWER DEVELOPMENT: Task 3: Interval Exercise
Task 4: Continuous Exercise

**Figure 6.1**

a "roller coaster" pattern, fluctuating quite drastically from its low to high points (see Figure 6.1). A walk (three minutes)-jog (one minute) exercise program is a classic example of interval conditioning; whereas walking and jogging at a set pace are continuous in nature.

Research findings* indicate that interval exercise is more efficient and less fatiguing than the continuous methods. Exercise physiologists speculate that the periods of low intensity

*E. Fox and D. Mathews, *Interval Training: Conditioning for Sports and General Fitness* (Philadelphia: W. B. Saunders, 1974).

physical activity incorporated into the interval workout allow locomotive and service organs to be replenished with needed metabolites, thus warding off their buildup of debilitating waste products. It would be wise to keep this in mind not only when constructing an aerobic conditioning program, but also during the performance of required occupational or home related exercise duties including gardening, car waxing, snow shoveling, and housework. They may take a longer time to complete, but you will definitely accomplish all muscular work tasks with a greater degree of effectiveness and safety when you perform them intermittently.

In continuous exercise for aerobic power development, heart rate must be sustained within the predetermined target zone throughout the body portion of the workout. For interval conditioning programs designed for the same purpose, the heart rate is made to rise above the target point during the heavy work period. Timewise, it could range from one and one-half to five minutes in duration compared to the lighter intensity exercise interval which typically lasts thirty seconds to three minutes. This is clearly illustrated in Figure 6.1.

Action sports (like basketball, soccer, hockey, handball, squash, and tennis) and many dance activities are, by their very

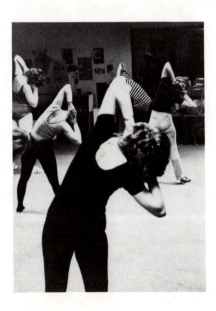

nature, interval exercise. However, they are neither as well controlled nor as potentially effective in outcome as more structured interval walking, jogging, running, swimming, or cycling programs.

Advanced or high level aerobic power exercise programs, it must be remembered, create the most severe degree of service network stress known to human beings. Such regimens are suited to highly fit individuals such as those conditioning for the rigors of athletic competition. They are not (I repeat NOT!) geared for previously sedentary people, young or old, with lower levels of aerobic fitness. Finally, attempts to improve aerobic endurance for low to moderate intensity exercise tasks might best precede those designed to elevate aerobic power.

# MAJOR AEROBIC PHYSICAL ACTIVITIES: PROS AND CONS

The pros and cons of the most popular aerobic physical activities are outlined in Table 6.3 below. Basically, they are performed in either a continuous or interval manner and for purposes of aerobic endurance or power benefits.

## TRADITIONAL AEROBIC CONDITIONING ACTIVITIES

Walking, jogging, swimming, cycling, rope skipping, and calisthenics have been utilized for years as aerobic conditioners. They lend themselves to simple exercise program design and can be geared with little complication to people of the lowest to the highest fitness capacities. For these physical activities, dosage increments in line with fitness improvement are easily incorporated. Participant performance improvement in them is also readily ascertained. Much of their popularity (with the exception of swimming) lies in their meager requirements (movement skills, facilities, and equipment) and the fact that

## Table 6.3

## Summarization of Features of Popular Aerobic Physical Activities

| Physical Activity | Performance Hints | Positive Features | Negative Features |
|---|---|---|---|
| Walking and Pace Walking | • Walk with good posture; pull shoulders back, keep back straight, and try to keep chest lifted.<br>• Tighten mid-section muscles and keep pelvis under spine (for back-ache prevention).<br>• Walk briskly enough to activate service network to desired level.<br>• Hill climbing is challenging. It is encouraged because it magnifies the degree of service network activation.<br>• Some pace walkers can actually travel faster than many joggers. | • Most common form of exercise because it is both practical and convenient. Can be performed almost any place, at any time, without special equipment. No complex movement skills necessary.<br>• Less traumatic to weight-bearing joints than jogging and most action sports performed in upright position; thus, injury risk is reduced.<br>• Ideal activity for poorly fit who desire to develop aerobic endurance and to control obesity.<br>• Requires as much energy expenditure per mile as jogging at moderate pace (5-11 mph). | • May find it relaxing, but many feel it is boring, unchallenging, and non-competitive.<br>• Must walk long distance to be of fitness value.<br>• Although same energy expenditure as jogging at moderate pace, one can jog a greater distance in much shorter time period than by walking. |
| Jogging | • Utilize good posture as in walking.<br>• Be certain weight-bearing body parts are in good repair to sustain shock they must bear.<br>• Jogging on soft surfaces (e.g., grass) is less stressful to the joints than on harder surfaces. Beware, however, of safety hazards such as rocks, crevices, uneven clumps of grass, holes, hidden debris, etc.<br>• Stretch out upper and lower leg muscles and heel tendons after jogging. | • Like walking, a very practical and convenient physical activity.<br>• Can jog a greater distance in set time period than would have been covered by walking, resulting in higher energy expenditure potential.<br>• Excellent for weight control.<br>• Excellent for both aerobic power and endurance development. | • Severe stress (pounding) to weight-bearing joints of locomotive network. Foot can strike ground 1000 times per mile, each with force of three times that of body weight. Can cause (or aggravate) a host of debilitating joint conditions (see Chapter 9).<br>• Can lead to imbalance in muscle development of legs.<br>• Can produce tightness in leg musculature and knee joint inflexibility. |

*(continued)*

## Table 6.3 *(continued)*

| Physical Activity | Performance Hints | Positive Features | Negative Features |
|---|---|---|---|
| Swimming | • Swim goggles prevent eye irritation from salt water and chemically treated water.<br>• Swimming skills performed in back position should be used often for those who find breathing a problem when swimming in the face-forward position. | • Probably best overall type of aerobic exercise. Least traumatic to locomotive system, since performed in horizontal position in weightless conditions within water.<br>• Especially appropriate for heavier people and those with orthopedic problems and handicaps.<br>• Energy expenditure is four times greater than walking and jogging the same distance.<br>• Practically no chance of body overheating when performed during warm weather.<br>• Merely submerging the body in water improves blood circulation. Even poorly skilled and handicapped persons can derive aerobic benefits from performance of basic movements (calisthenics, running, hopping, etc.) in water. | • Major requisites for participation in swimming conditioning program include adequate swimming skills and access to supervised facility.<br>• Although energy expenditure is greater than walking and jogging same distance, it takes a considerably longer period of time to swim that distance than to walk or jog it. |
| Sports | • Try to develop interests and skills in sports you can perform for the rest of your life.<br>• Conditioning for stressful sports is often warranted since it can aid in effective and safe performance.<br>• Progressive stretching of locomotive body parts utilized in performance of sport skills is recommended before and after participation. | • Potentially the most popular and enjoyable mode of aerobic exercise for most people. More inviting for those of you who do not care for solitary, repetitive aspects of the likes of walking, jogging, swimming, etc.<br>• Great many sports from which to choose with a wide range of potential service network activation from the very light (e.g. golf) to the exhaustive (X-country skiing).<br>• Most are interval in nature. | • Many aspects of sports are inherently dangerous to locomotive network and other body areas.<br>• Often require specialized skills, equipment, and facilities.<br>• Team sports necessitate the recruitment of other players.<br>• Lesser degree of control over intensity of energy demand than more typical aerobic conditioning tasks.<br>• Can cause imbalance in development of muscles and joints. |

*(continued)*

## Table 6.3 (continued)

| Physical Activity | Performance Hints | Positive Features | Negative Features |
|---|---|---|---|
| Calisthenics and Circuit Training* | • Use a well rounded core of calisthenics for total body development (see basic core of calisthenic activities presented in Chapter 7, pp. 134-138).<br>• Listening, to music while performing can make these exercise programs less tedious and more enjoyable. | • Could very well be the most practical of all physical activities with few time, weather, facility, or equipment requisites.<br>• Major fitness benefit is muscle endurance development, but if calisthenic tasks are performed in succession of one another for over five minutes, heart rate can be elevated sufficiently to improve aerobic efficiency. | • Many persons find these activities unchallenging, boring, tedious, and unexciting. |
| Cycling | • Safety is a must! Stay away from traffic congested areas.<br>• Be careful at all times to avoid collisions with pedestrians, automobiles, and other cycles.<br>• Stretch out lower extremities before and after cycling workouts. | • Long distance cycling is growing in popularity as both a competitive sport and leisure exercise pursuit.<br>• Excellent means of service network activation.<br>• Performed in sitting (non-weight bearing) position. Develops lower extremity muscles and joints and aerobic efficiency without the pounding and stress to feet and knees. | • Must have bicycle and safe riding area.<br>• Can be dangerous! Accident rate for cyclists is on the rise.<br>• Stress to rectum. Known to cause or aggravate rectal problems, especially among long distance riders.<br>• Can cause overdevelopment of lower extremities and underdevelopment of upper body areas. |
| Rope Skipping | • Listening to music and acquisition of a variety of rope skipping techniques can relieve potential monotony of this exercise. | • Very practical and inexpensive activity.<br>• Excellent aerobic activity. Simultaneous use of arms and legs can produce moderate to high energy output, thus providing adequate service network activation. | • Very repetitious, monotonous, and boring for many individuals.<br>• Effective jumping skills required.<br>• Can be stressful to feet and ankles. |
| Dancing | • Should be performed on regular basis to reap aerobic benefits.<br>• Other forms of aerobic conditioning can supplement dance workouts. | • Traditional (ballet, folk, square, and ballroom) and new forms of dance such as aerobic dancing provide aerobic benefits as well as fun and enjoyment. | • Dance skills required.<br>• Can involve fees for practice sessions and travel to and from performance facilities.<br>• Often performed only at designated times and/or under supervision of dance instructor. |

*Circuit training is discussed in Chapter 7.

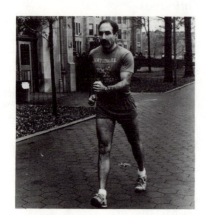
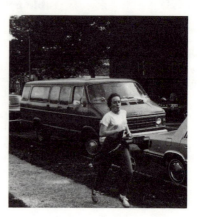
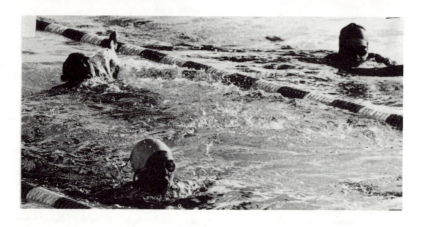
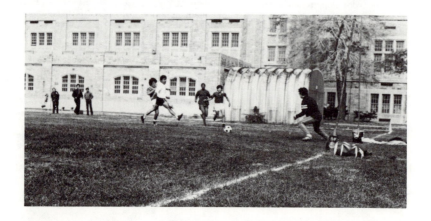

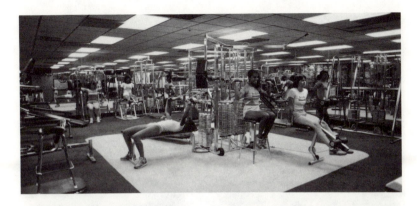

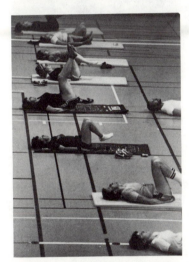

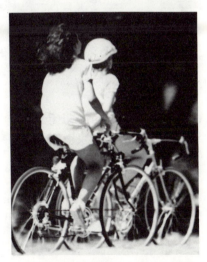

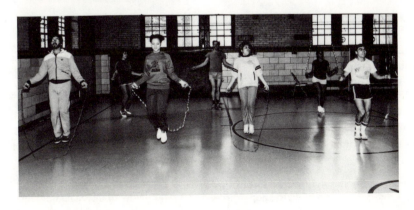

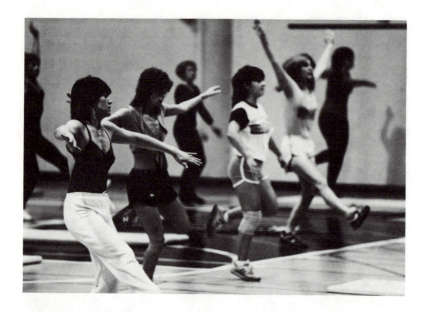

they can be performed alone or with others at any time of day, the year round. Sports and dance activities, on the other hand, usually do require substantially more in the way of skills, participant fees, and special equipment and facilities.

An example of an aerobic endurance walk-jog program which can be performed continuously or intermittently is presented in Table 6.4. As indicated, you initiate it at any of four

### Table 6.4

### Elementary Walk-Jog Aerobic Endurance Exercise Program

| Aerobic Efficiency Fitness Rating* | Intensity** | Duration (min.) | Frequency (Times/wk.) |
|---|---|---|---|
| Poor | Slow to Fast Walk | 8-20 | 2-4 |
| Moderate | Fast Walk-Slow Jog | 15-30 | 3-5 |
| Good to Excellent | Slow to Moderate Jog | > 30 | > 4 |

*Determine rating through procedures in Chapter 4.
**These intensities are intended to keep exercise heart rates below 70% of maximum heart rate.

**Table 6.5**

## Continuous Walking-Jogging Exercise Program for Aerobic Power

| Aerobic Fitness Rating* | Intensity Target Heart Rate (% of HR max) | Duration (min.) | Frequency (Times/wk.) |
|---|---|---|---|
| Low | 70 | 10-20 | 3 |
| Moderate | 71-80 | 20-30 | 4-5 |
| Excellent | 81-90 | > 30 | > 5 — to twice daily |

*As indicated by results of appraisals attained in Chapter 4.

different dosage levels depending on your state of aerobic efficiency. Tables 6.5 and 6.6 represent basic continuous and interval aerobic power exercise programs. Keep in mind that similar formats manipulating major dosage variables could be

**Table 6.6**

## Interval Running Program for Aerobic Power*

| Distance | 400 yards |
|---|---|
| Time** | 1½-3 minutes |
| Rest Interval - Light jogging | 1-2 minutes |
| Reps (repetition of above distance)** | 3-5 |
| Sets** | 1-3 |
| Frequency (times/week) | 3-5 |

*This type of exercise program is intended for people with good to excellent aerobic efficiency.

**As the program is continued, these dosage variables can be manipulated to make workouts longer and more intense. Start with one set of three repetitions and proceed toward the completion of three sets of five repetitions.

utilized for cycling, swimming, and rope skipping programs designed for the same purposes.

Many fitness advocates, including myself, feel that swimming is one of the best all-around conditioning activities. Not only does it lend itself to effective aerobic development, but it tends to enhance the fitness of critical locomotive areas of the body without pounding or jolting them. Examples of aerobic swimming regimens are presented in Table 6.7.

## Table 6.7

## Aerobic Swimming Programs

### A. Aerobic Endurance Swimming Program*

| Aerobic Efficiency | Swim Speed** | Duration (minutes) | Frequency (Times/week) |
|---|---|---|---|
| Low | Very | < 15 | 2-3 |
| Average | Slow to | 16-30 | 3-5 |
| Excellent | Moderate | > 30 | > 5 |

*Can be performed intermittently or continuously.
**Exercise HR should remain below 70% of maximum heart rate.

### B. Interval Swimming Program*

| | |
|---|---|
| Distance | 100 yards |
| Time | 2-3 minutes |
| Rest Interval (resting stroke) | 1-2 minutes |
| Reps | 5-8 |
| Sets | 1-3 |
| Frequency (times/week) | 2-6 |

*Exercise HR should be made to climb to 70% of maximum HR or above.

## PREPARATION FOR LONG DISTANCE AEROBIC PERFORMANCE EVENTS

Many individuals have come to enjoy, in recent days, the challenge of long distance road, cycling, and swimming events. What must be both recognized and realized by them is that the conditioning for, as well as the actual competition of such long distance events, are very stressful to the locomotive and service networks of the body. Unfortunately, a great number of these exercise enthusiasts are not fully conditioned to the degree required for such competition, and they suffer the consequences in terms of injury and debilitation. Table 6.8 reflects the type of exercise preparation (in weekly mileage) required to ready a runner for a safe completion of a half-marathon and marathon road race.

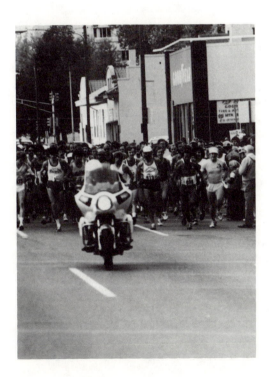

**Table 6.8**

**Preparatory Conditioning Schedule for
Long Distance Road Races**

| | Weekly Mileage Required | |
|---|---|---|
| | Half-Marathon | Marathon |
| Time Prior to Event | (13.1 miles) | (26.2 miles) |
| 3-5 Months Before | > 40 | > 60 |
| 2 Months Before | > 30 | > 50 |
| | Plus two 7-9 mile runs; two weeks apart | Plus two 15-20 mile runs; two weeks apart |
| 1 Month Before | Taper to 20 | Taper to 40 |
| 2 Weeks Before | Taper to 10-15: (Last 7-mile run) | Taper to 14-20: (Last 10-mile run) |
| 2 Days before Event | Rest or light jogging | |

## DANCE AND COMPETITIVE SPORTS

Dance activities and sports are ever growing in popularity among people around the globe. Most of us seldom give recognition to dance as a potential physical fitness producer. However, the overall energy requirements of ballet and theatrical dancing are most extensive, and those who regularly perform them usually possess exceptionally high levels of aerobic power as well as flexibility, strength, and endurance. Observation also indicates envied states of leanness among dancers who perform professionally.

Disco dancing can also be quite strenuous, while folk, ballroom, and square dancing are generally lighter in intensity. In short, the author advocates all forms of dance as potential fitness activities for those with interests and the ability to perform them.

Aerobic dancing techniques, originated by Jackie Sorensen, continue to gain new advocates, including males. A typical aerobic dance routine incorporates a combination of repetitive dance steps, stretching motions, and other simple movements performed to popular music. Most participants find the aerobic dance workout so enjoyable, they hardly realize they are exercising. The Sorensen aerobic dance program is conducted twice weekly for eight weeks. Each session is conducted for a period of 50-60 minutes during which warm-up precedes and cool-down follows the more stressful dance routines. Target heart rates are determined for each participant; after each routine, heart rates are measured by performers to see if they are in the target zone. If well above or below the target, the dancer is instructed to slow or accelerate the movements in the next dance. The weekly dance routines are progressively intensified in demands and thus should provide for development of aerobic capacity as well as improvement in flexibility and endurance in major muscle-joint areas.

The negative features of aerobic dance programs are: enrollment in the program usually involves a monetary fee; the services of a dance leader are required; and the program is conducted in a special facility to and from which one must travel. Similar drawbacks exist for other dance activities but more so for ballet and theatrical dance, which also have a more sophisticated level of dance skills as a performance requisite.

Sports represent the major means through which people of all nations engage in recreational exercise. Their energy demands range from the light (e.g., bowling) to the exhaustive (cross-country skiing). Systematic participation in moderate to heavy intensity sports such as basketball, handball, racquetball, soccer, squash, tennis, volleyball, and skiing can contribute to aerobic fitness. Basically, the greater the sport's energy demands, the greater the taxation of the service networks. Light intensity sports are more suited for aerobic endurance purposes, whereas the more strenuous ones can be considered aerobic power development sports.

For the most part, sports and dance are more appropriate activities for the maintenance rather than the development of fitness. In fact, many athletes and dancers, both professional and amateur, have come to recognize the value of supplementary conditioning programs as significant requisites to effective performance, injury prevention, and to the body's overall capacity to meet the requirements of sports and dance.

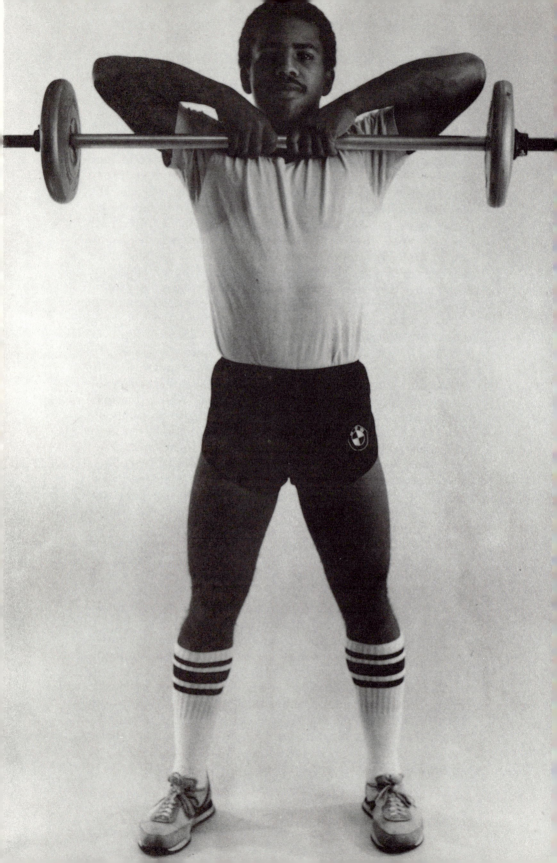

# Chapter Seven

# PHYSICAL ACTIVITY PROGRAMS FOR LOCOMOTIVE NETWORK EFFICIENCY

*"What a disgrace it is for a man to grow old
without ever seeing the beauty and strength of
which his body is capable."*

*Socrates*

---

**KEY WORDS**

| | |
|---|---|
| Core | Calisthenics |
| Set | Isometrics |
| Reps | Isokinetics |
| Static Stretching | Circuit Training |

---

## GENERAL INFORMATION CONCERNING EXERCISE FOR LOCOMOTIVE NETWORK EFFICIENCY

All the body movements that you make are direct responses to activation of specific muscles, bones, and joints. Progressive resistance, repetition, and stretching exercise programs represent the best means of developing the qualities of fitness associated with locomotive network efficiency, namely, strength, endurance, and flexibility (Chapter 3). As we commence this discussion of the major ways to promote these qualities, two rather relevant points of information warrant reinforcement. First is the fact that the locomotive network is extensive — with many critical parts of it in need of development. Second is the reality that the fitness quality attained within a particular locomotive area is specific to the modes of physical activity that you perform (Chapter 5).

Repetitive movements of most forms of aerobic exercise tend to elevate the endurance of muscles and joints they activate to the neglect of other significant ones that are not utilized. For example, jogging, cycling, and sports performed in the upright position enhance the endurance capacity of the anterior thigh and calf (back of lower leg) muscles. Yet, they fail to develop the musculature of the posterior thigh and anterior lower leg regions and involve minimum activation of midsectional and upper extremity muscles. Nor do they promote joint flexibility. The fact of the matter is that they are more likely to produce the opposite effect, that is, joint stiffness and muscle tightness in the lower extremities.

The modes of physical activity presented in this chapter are worth learning and practicing because they can result in the development and maintenance of strength, endurance, and flexibility in the more critical areas of your body. In the construction of all such programs, **an exercise core or group of movement tasks** is selected, each stressing a different muscle-joint locality. The core exercises chosen should be ones that develop weak muscles and inflexible joints. However, in the absence of specific weaknesses and limitations, a core of varied exercises that utilize the major muscles and joints of the upper and lower extremities, mid-section, and spine would be warranted.

An exercise core, generally designed to include some five to fifteen different movement tasks, is usually performed more than once. **The term "set" refers to each separate completion of the entire exercise core, while the number of times each movement task is repeated during a set is defined as "rep" (repetition).** For example, you might design an exercise program that calls for a core of eight different movements that are performed in three sets of ten reps. This basic system is incorporated in all progressive resistive, repetition, and stretching regimens.

Let's examine each type of exercise program in greater detail.

# PROGRESSIVE STRETCHING

The author believes that the most relevant form of locomotive network exercise is progressive stretching. Probably no fitness outcome is more neglected than is joint flexibility. The regular practice of body movements that increase joint angles by stretching your muscles, tendons, and ligaments enhances flexibility as well as producing other potential benefits (Table 7.1).

### Table 7.1

### Potential Benefits of Progressive Stretching Exercise Programs

- Improved joint flexibility.
- Proper posture and body carriage.
- Stability of joints and muscles in resisting stresses of movement (reduced risk of injuries such as sprains and strains as noted in Chapter 9).
- Improved circulation within internal organs.
- A general feeling of well-being and relaxation (euphoria).

Structural limitations within critical joints and muscles often predispose an individual to poor flexibility. Failure to stretch soft muscle-joint tissues regularly can only add to their lack of elasticity. And, to reiterate what was mentioned earlier in the chapter, the repetitive movements of most physical activities often precipitate muscle-joint tightening.

Hundreds of valuable stretching tasks exist. Hatha yoga is an example of a currently popular program of progressive (elementary to advanced) stretches. It is highly recommended for all, but especially for those of you who have a tendency toward tight muscles and stiff joints. Stretching movements could (and should) also be incorporated with little difficulty as one of the components of your regular exercise routines.

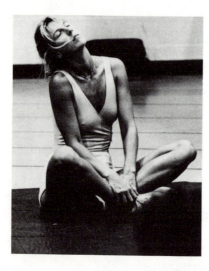

Hatha yoga

Stretching, a form of negative muscular work, does not involve waste production within activated muscle tissues. Thus, it can be performed daily with minimum threat to any inability to recover from it. The duration of a full hatha yoga or other flexibility-type workout will depend, obviously, on the number of stretches included in the exercise core. Ideally, two sets of core stretching tasks should be performed, each set involving two reps.

## WHEN AND HOW TO STRETCH

You may recall that the soft tissues of muscles, tendons, and joints are more elastic when they are heated. Whenever you stretch, by all means first warm up your body and loosen locomotive tissues through progressively light to moderate aerobic and calisthenic tasks for a minimum of eight minutes.

When performing two sets of stretches, execute the first with restraint (submaximally). The second set can then be executed with close to maximum stretching capacity when locomotive organs are more receptive to it. Concerning when to stretch, one final recommendation must be emphasized to those of you who include a vigorous stretching routine within your warm-up period prior to embarking in more extensive physical activity. **Contrary to such practice, the more appropriate time to perform this routine is after heavier activity, when fully heated soft tissues are more elastic and ready for maximum stretching.** Post-exercise stretching is also believed to be conducive to the recuperation of joints and locomotive tissues previously activated.

All stretching movements should be executed slowly and gradually. The stretched position, once attained, can be held for a minimum of twelve seconds and should not cause a severe degree of pain. This is referred to as a **static stretch** and is preferable to **ballistic stretching** which involves lunging, jerking, or bouncing. Such motions are a greater threat to the tearing of your soft muscle-joint tissues and are not as effective as static stretching in the promotion of permanent joint flexibility.

The breath should not be held during a static stretch. Air should be inhaled and exhaled in a slow, relaxed manner. A state of overall calmness and relaxation in other body parts ("differential relaxation") should be maintained as you progress toward and hold the stretched position desired. Rather than dwell on any discomfort that might be felt, you should close your eyes and focus the mind on the continuation of slow, easy breathing.

# CALISTHENICS

Movements of body parts in opposition to resistive forces tend to promote strength and endurance. **Calisthenics, ele-**

Comparison of Two Persons Performing Chin-ups

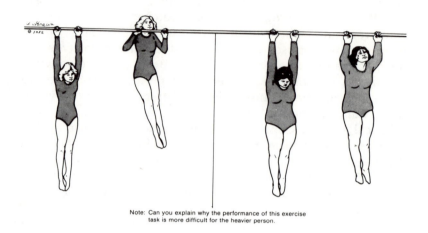

Note: Can you explain why the performance of this exercise
task is more difficult for the heavier person.

**Figure 7.1**

**mentary movements made against gravity,** are executed in the upright, sitting, and lying positions. In performing them, resistance is dependent on the relative weight of the particular body area being moved. For example, in chinning, the total body weight is the actual resistance. The tension created within the upper arm muscles (biceps) provides the actual pulling force that causes the elbows to bend as the body is raised up from the hanging position. Evidently, the upper arm muscle tension required to complete a chin is considerably greater for a heavy person than for one of normal weight (see Figure 7.1).

Regarding dosage manipulation for calisthenics, the resistances generally remain constant while the exercise core, sets, and reps are subject to variation. Table 7.2 represents a typical calisthenic exercise routine. This and other calisthenic regimens will generate muscle-joint endurance rather than strength or flexibility, since they incorporate progressive repetition rather than resistance increments. As is the case with stretching movements, there are numerous valuable calisthenics advocated by different fitness authorities. A series of the more relevant ones (in conjunction with important stretches) are presented on pages 143-145.

## Table 7.2

## Calisthenic Exercise Routine

**General Directions:** Perform one to three sets of the calisthenic core, starting with the lowest reps. When lowest reps can be performed for three sets, gradually increase reps toward maximum number indicated for each calisthenic task.

| Body Area Activated | Calisthenic Core | Reps | Sets |
|---|---|---|---|
| Ankle, feet and posterior lower leg | Heel Raise | 15-40 | 1-3 |
| Anterior thigh and knee | Half Squats | 10-40 | 1-3 |
| Mid-Section | Bent Knee Sit-up | 3-15 | 1-3 |
| Sides of Waist and hip | Single Side Leg Raise (Right) | 5-20 | 1-3 |
| | Single Side Leg Raise (Left) | 5-20 | 1-3 |
| Lower Back and hip | Single Prone Leg Raise (Left) | 5-15 | 1-3 |
| | Single Prone Leg Raise (Right) | 5-15 | 1-3 |
| Anterior upper arm, shoulder, elbow, and wrist | Chin | 2-8 | 1-3 |
| Posterior upper arm, chest, shoulder, elbow, and wrist | Push-up | 3-15 | 1-3 |

# WEIGHT TRAINING

Progressive overload in weight training* can be administered through elevations in either resistance (load) or reps. **In**

*Weight training is not the same as weight lifting, which is a competitive sport involving a variety of strength and power maneuvers.

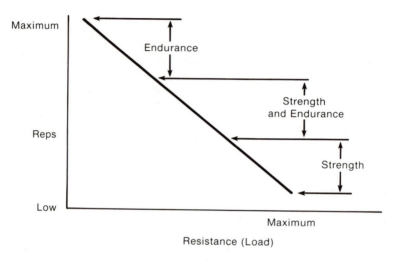

Relationship between Resistance and Reps in
the Development of Strength and Endurance

Note: Low resistance, high rep exercise results in endurance
improvement; whereas high resistance, low rep exercise
is more suited to gains in strength.

**Figure 7.2**

line with a basic physiologic principle, low reps-high resistance
conditioning fosters strength development; whereas high reps-
low resistance weight training tends to produce endurance (see
Figure 7.2).

Rapid motions against moderate to maximum resistances
lead more to power production. Table 7.3 presents a simplified
set of procedures to be incorporated in the construction of
weight training programs designed for strength (Prescription A)
and endurance (Prescription B).

A core of basic weight training movements that you could
easily execute with conventional barbells, dumbells, and more
recently developed resistance apparatus (e.g., universal machine
as pictured in photograph ) is presented on pages 146-153.

## Table 7.3

## Basic Weight Training Procedures

1. Select a core of five or more weight training tasks.
2. After a minimum eight minute warm-up, determine for each task selected, an **approximate** maximum resistance that could be lifted once through full range of motion. Record this number.
3. To determine suitable weight resistances, reps, and sets, follow either Prescription A or B.

### Prescription A: Strength Program

- Calculate starting weight resistance by subtracting the following weights from the maximum resistances for one lift:

| Maximum Resistance in Lbs. for One Lift | Lbs. Subtracted |
|:---:|:---:|
| $< 30$ | 5 |
| 31-50 | 10 |
| 51-80 | 15 |
| 81-100 | 20 |
| $> 100$ | 30 |

- Starting sets: 2
  Starting reps $< 5$
- Work toward completing 3 sets of 5 reps. When accomplished, increase weight resistance 5-10 lbs. and start again.

### Prescription B: Endurance Program

- Calculate starting weight resistances by taking 1/5 to 1/3 of maximum resistance for one lift.
- Starting sets: 2
  Starting reps $< 16$
- Work toward the execution of 3 sets of 15 reps. When accomplished, add 2½-10 lbs. and start again.

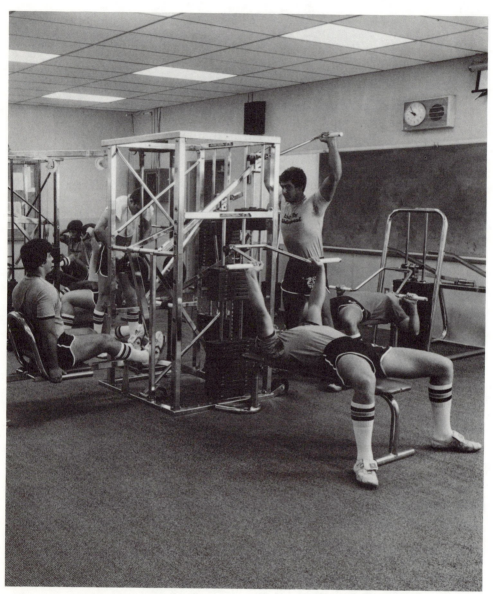

The Universal Machine.

Courtesy of Universal,
P.O. Box 1270, Cedar
Rapids, Iowa 52406.

# ISOMETRICS

**An isometric movement is one that is attempted against an immovable resistance.** The angle of the joint is usually reduced to a set degree within its normal range of motion. The extent of this motion relates directly to the level of shortening that takes place within the muscle group activating the joint; that is, your muscle proceeds to contract to a certain length despite the continued elevation in its tension buildup. It is recommended that the gradual buildup and return from maximum tension in the partial state of contraction occur over an 8-15 second period.

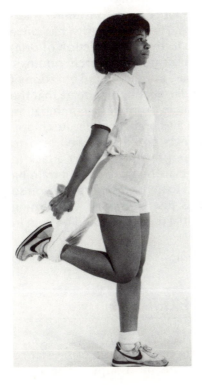

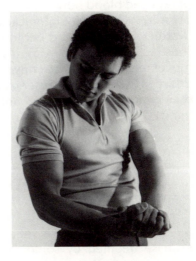

*This page and page 128:* Students performing popular isometric exercise tasks

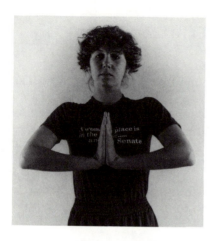

Isometric exercises gained recognition in the 1950s when researchers reported that gains in muscle strength and endurance from short bouts of isometric training equaled or surpassed those attained through the more time consuming traditional weight training procedures. Their popularity has since declined markedly, however, due to the contradiction of original supportive evidence by subsequent research findings. Critics of this training technique have also raised the question of its potential danger to cardiovascular health. It appears that the performance of isometric movements produces a combination of reduced blood flow to the heart and brain and elevates blood pressure. These physiological effects could very well lead to dizziness, fainting, and could even precipitate heart attack in those susceptible to it. Almost any calisthenic or weight training movement can easily be converted to an isometric task if you so desire. However, the reservations just expressed concerning their overrated benefits and potential dangers should be kept in mind.

## ISOKINETIC EXERCISE

**Isokinetic exercise** is yet another recent form of resistance exercise deemed by some to be the most superior to date.

Specialized devices such as the popular *Nautilus* machine are requisite to the performance of isokinetics.

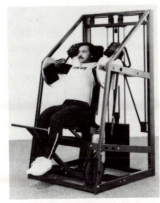

The Nautilus Machine

There are several features of calisthenics and weight training movements that limit their overall physiological effectiveness. While not advocated, they can be executed with great speed, causing the buildup of momentum to actually contribute to movement production. This is especially true during the return of limbs to their starting position via muscle lengthening and tension release, more technically referred to as the eccentric phase of movement. Joints are all too often not made to move through their full range of motion during our completion of typical calisthenic and weight training tasks. **In performing isokinetics, the level of resistance is made to equal the level of tension created throughout the movement.** Isokinetic tasks are also completed slowly through their full range of motion, starting from prestretched positions. Momentum is virtually eliminated even when returning to your starting position.

For isokinetic routines, strength is said to respond best to three sets of two-three reps of the movement task. Regarding frequency, the routine would be completed on alternate days.

Even if the claim for its superiority were true, a primary requisite for participation in isokinetic exercise programs is accessibility to a *Nautilus* or other expensive, sophisticated device. More often than not, such pieces of machinery are not going to be available to the average, everyday exerciser. Another drawback is that you must learn how to set and use these devices properly.

# CIRCUIT TRAINING

**Circuit training** is a potentially excellent type of exercise program for balanced fitness development. A well-constructed circuit training regimen conditions your major muscles and joints while fostering aerobic efficiency. Demands are placed on the service network because you attempt to complete the circuit exercise tasks in as short a time period as possible.

The two major concerns in setting up a circuit program are the selection of the circuit exercises and the target time. **A circuit generally involves a core of exercise tasks performed sequentially in three sets of varying reps.** Calisthenic, stretching, and weight training circuits can easily be constructed. The number of minutes allotted for the completion of the circuit is referred to as the **target time.**

For the sample calisthenic circuit regimen presented in Table 7.4, you would select a suitable starting circuit level ranging from A-D. Record the time it takes to execute the entire circuit (three sets of required reps) and subtract two minutes from it. This becomes your target time. Subsequently, when you can complete the circuit within the target time, proceed to the next reps level.

Circuits also can be self-designed rather easily. To do so, you would first select a suitable core of tasks to include in your circuit and then attempt to execute as many reps as possible for each circuit task selected in a set time ranging from 15-60 seconds. (Provide yourself a 1-2 minute rest period between the timed performance of each circuit task.) After finishing the testing and the recording of reps, the circuit load is determined by taking one-half or three-quarters of the reps completed for each circuit task performed. The self-designed circuit program is finalized by calculating the target time, which is done by adding all the testing times and multiplying this number by three. The above procedures are demonstrated in Table 7.5.

In performing the circuit, the first set should be completed with little difficulty because it is well below the maximum capability of the performer. However, overload tends to commence during the latter stages of the second set and throughout the third set when you approach your near maximum endurance capacity for each circuit task. Progressive dosage incre-

## Table 7.4

## Calisthenic Circuit Training Regimen

| Calisthenic Tasks | | | | Target Time: _____ | |
|---|---|---|---|---|---|
| | | | Reps | | |
| | Level: | A | B | C | D |
| Poco Hops | | 10 | 15 | 25 | 40 |
| Shoulder Rolls | | 10 | 15 | 25 | 40 |
| Jumping Jacks | | 10 | 15 | 25 | 40 |
| Half Squats | | 8 | 10 | 15 | 25 |
| Heel Raises | | 10 | 15 | 20 | 25 |
| Knee-ups | | 3 | 5 | 8 | 12 |
| Bent Knee sit-ups | | 3 | 5 | 10 | 20 |
| Modified push-ups | | 3 | 5 | 8 | 12 |
| Single Side Leg Raises (Right) | | 8 | 10 | 15 | 20 |
| Single Side Leg Raises (Left) | | 8 | 10 | 15 | 20 |
| Single Prone Leg Raises (Right) | | 3 | 5 | 8 | 12 |
| Single Prone Leg Raises (Left) | | 3 | 5 | 8 | 12 |

**General Directions:**

- Select suitable starting level (A-D).
- Complete three sets of calisthenic tasks at that level.
- Record time and subtract two minutes from it to determine target time.
- When capable of executing circuit in target time, proceed to next level.

ments can take place by: (a) decreasing the target time, (b) increasing the reps for circuit tasks, (c) completing the circuit (three sets) more than once during a workout, and (d) performing the circuit with greater frequency over the course of the week.

**One concluding note deserves mention regarding calisthenics, weight training, and circuit training. The movement tasks incorporated in these programs should stress all the major muscles associated with a particular joint as opposed to just one**

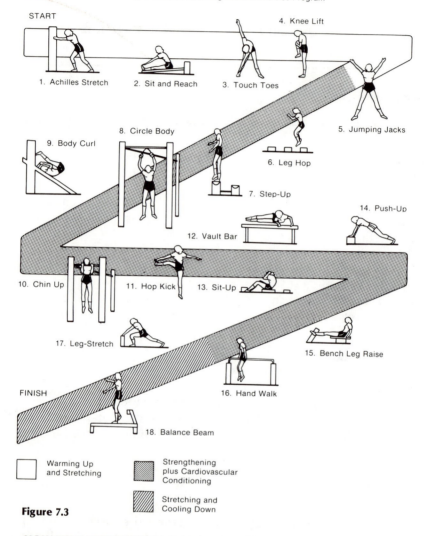

A Self-Guided Parcourse Circuit: Combination Calisthenic-Stretching Circuit and Walk-Jog Aerobic Exercise Program

START

4. Knee Lift

1. Achilles Stretch    2. Sit and Reach    3. Touch Toes

5. Jumping Jacks

8. Circle Body

9. Body Curl

6. Leg Hop

7. Step-Up

14. Push-Up

12. Vault Bar

10. Chin Up    11. Hop Kick    13. Sit-Up

17. Leg-Stretch

15. Bench Leg Raise

FINISH

16. Hand Walk

18. Balance Beam

☐ Warming Up and Stretching

▦ Strengthening plus Cardiovascular Conditioning

▨ Stretching and Cooling Down

**Figure 7.3**

## HOW THE PARCOURSE FITNESS CIRCUIT WORKS:

Parcourse fitness circuits are designed for people of every fitness level. Spaced throughout a walking-jogging course, are a series of exercise stations marked by parcourse signs. At each station, as directed by sign illustrations and instructions, you perform a specific stretching or calisthenic task. Each station also provides suggested numbers of reps for each level of fitness (e.g. starting, sporting, and championship). When completed, you walk, jog, or run to the next station where another exercise task is presented. One completed circuit represents a balance workout for your entire body. Best of all, it is individualized, because you set the pace.

## Table 7.5

## Self-Designed Calisthenics Circuit Training Program

| Circuit Exercise | Test Time (15-60 sec.) | Total Reps | ½ or ¾ Reps | Performance Record Date | Time |
|---|---|---|---|---|---|
| 1. Poco Hops | 1 min. | 40 | 20 | ———— | ———— |
| 2. Shoulder Rolls | 30 secs. | 40 | 30 | ———— | ———— |
| 3. Jumping Jacks | 1 min. | 50 | 25 | ———— | ———— |
| 4. Half Squats | 30 secs. | 18 | 9 | ———— | ———— |
| 5. Heel Raises | 30 secs. | 35 | 27 | ———— | ———— |
| 6. Single Side Leg Raise (Right) | 45 secs. | 20 | 10 | ———— | ———— |
| 7. Single Side Leg Raise (Left) | 45 secs. | 21 | 10 | ———— | ———— |
| 8. Bent Knee Sit-ups | 30 secs. | 16 | 8 | ———— | ———— |
| 9. Modified Push-ups | 15 secs. | 8 | 4 | ———— | ———— |
| 10. Knee-ups | 15 secs. | 7 | 4 | ———— | ———— |
| 11. | | | | ———— | ———— |
| 12. | | | | ———— | ———— |

Total Test Time (min.) $6 \times 3 = 18$ Target Time

**of them.** This will help to prevent excessive muscle tightening while promoting a balance in the strength-endurance capacities among muscles. These outcomes, in effect, should enhance the range of joint motion and reduce the chances of suffering a muscle strain.

# A BATTERY OF SIGNIFICANT LIFETIME CALISTHENIC AND STRETCHING TASKS

The exercise tasks pictured and described below, when practiced on a regular basis, can help you to develop and maintain an optimal level of locomotive network efficiency. They are basic calisthenic and stretching movements designed to: (a) enhance strength, endurance, and flexibility and (2) help prevent injury and infirmity within muscle-joint regions of your body.

Most of them can be modified to be made either less or more strenuous. Each should be executed to a degree that is in line with performer capability (readiness). In addition to how the exercise movement is completed, the number of sets and reps performed during a workout would also be determined individually.

# A. CALISTHENICS

### General Guidelines and Performance Hints

- Try to perform each calisthenic exercise slowly and through the fullest range of movement of which you are capable.
- Adequate strength to perform certain movement tasks might be lacking. Do not be discouraged if unable to perform a calisthenic fully. It will improve with practice. Modifications, when warranted, are also advocated to make more strenuous tasks less difficult to complete, while aiding in strength development of the muscles involved.
- Breathe naturally during the performance of each calisthenic.

### Side Leg Raise

**Purpose: For side of mid-section and hips.**
- Lie on the right side.

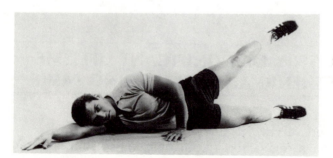

Side leg raise

- Position head on outstretched right arm and place left hand on floor in front of waist.
- Lift straightened left leg up as high as possible.
- Lower to starting position.
- After repeating desired number, turn to the left side and repeat with right leg.

**Double Leg Raise**

- More strenuous than single leg raise.
- Same procedure as above, except raise both legs simultaneously.

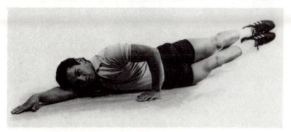

Double side leg raise

**Regular Bent Knee Sit-up**

**Purpose: For upper mid-section and to help correct or prevent lordosis and backache.**
- Assume supine (lying on back) position.
- Bend knees so that soles of feet are flat on the floor.
- Fold arms in front of chest.
- Pressing lower back down against the floor and tucking chin into the chest, curl up and touch elbows to the thigh.
- Return to starting position slowly.

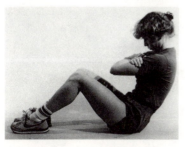

Regular bent knee sit-up

### Modified Sit-up

- To make less strenuous, place hands under thighs and help the curling movement by pulling with the arms.
- Can also be made less strenuous by anchoring the feet to the ground.

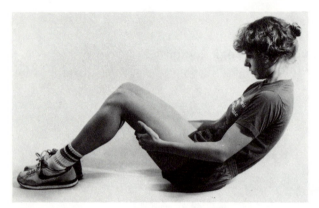

Modified
sit-up

**Note:** Some of you might have been taught to twist the spine as you perform the sit-up. This maneuver is to be avoided as it provides no extra benefit to the abdominal musculature, and can cause injury to the spinal column.

### Prone Leg Raise

**Purpose: For lower back (improve or prevent lordosis and low back pain).**
- Prone (lying face down) position with head turned to either side; cheek resting on back of hands folded under head.
- Raise left leg up, keeping the knee straight and the hips in contact with the ground.
- Lower to starting position slowly.
- Repeat with right leg.

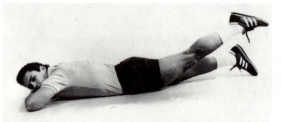

(Single)
prone
leg raise

### Double Prone Leg Raise

- More strenuous than single leg raise.
- Same directions as above, except raise both legs simultaneously.
- Spreading the legs after they are raised makes the task even more strenuous.

Double prone leg raise

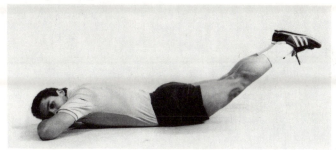

### Knee-up

**Purpose: For lower mid-section (helps correct or prevent abdominal sag, lordosis, and backache).**
- Supine position with knees bent and arms at the sides.
- Pressing lower back against the floor, bring the legs into the chest with the knees advancing toward the face.
- Return to starting position.

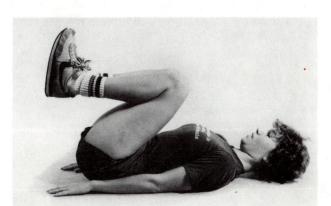

Knee-up

### Floor Push-up

**Purpose: For upper arms, shoulders, chest, and wrists.**
- Prone position with elbows bent and palms placed on the floor just outside of the shoulders.
- Keeping a straight line through the shoulders, hips, and ankles, push the body up to a fully extended elbow position.
- Lower to the floor, maintaining the straight body line.

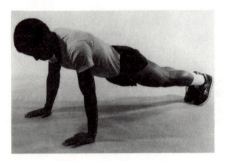

Floor push-up

### Modified Push-up

- To make less strenuous, modify by contacting the floor with bent knees rather than toes.
- In pushing up to the extended elbow position, keep straight line from shoulders to the knees.
- If lacking strength to push the body up in the modified position, constant repetition of lowering the straightened body from extended elbow position will help to develop that strength.

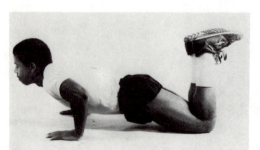

Modified push-up

# B. STATIC STRETCHING TASKS

### General Guidelines and Performance Hints

- Perform each movement slowly, with the stretching position held for 12-30 seconds.
- Avoid rapid lunging, jerking, or bouncing (can cause tissue tearing).
- Do not hold breath! Close your eyes and concentrate on slow, steady breathing as you move toward the degree of stretch desired (rather than on any discomfort experienced).
- Do not be discouraged if initial ability to stretch is limited. Practice will definitely bring improvement.
- Rest 5 to 10 seconds prior to repeating a stretching movement.

### Heel Cord Stretch

### Purpose: Heel cords (Achilles tendons) and calf (posterior lower leg) muscles.
- Face wall in standing position (at arm's length distance from wall).
- Keeping feet flat and back and legs straight, lean into wall by bending the elbows.
- Stretch can be increased by standing further from wall or by placing a book under balls of feet.

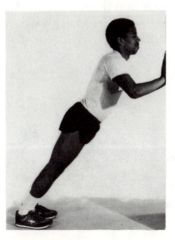

Heel cord stretch

### Sitting Straight Leg Reach (Hamstring Stretch)

**Purpose: Back of thighs, knee, and lower back.**
- Sit on floor with straight legs together and toes pointing upward.
- Bend at the waist with the back straight, head up, and keeping the legs completely straight, pull forward by grasping the lower legs with the hands as far down as you can reach.

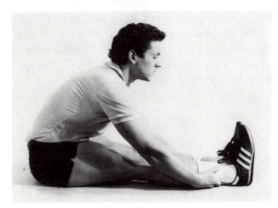

Sitting straight
leg reach

### Lying Bent Knee Thigh Stretch (Quads Stretch)

**Purpose: Anterior thigh and knee.**
- Sit on floor with right leg straight and left knee bent with inside lower left leg and ankle contacting floor.
- Grasp left ankle with left hand and lower torso backwards as far as possible toward full lying position.
- Perform with opposite leg.

Lying bent knee thigh stretch

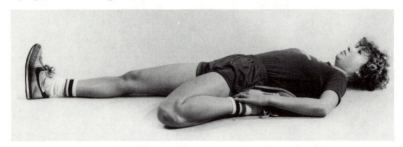

## Back Press

**Purpose: For pelvic area (help correct or prevent lordosis).**
- Supine position with knees bent and feet flat on floor.
- Pull in mid-section.
- (Tilt the pelvis forward) and try to press the lower back firmly against the floor.

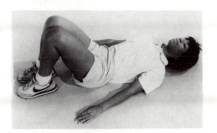

Back press

## Sitting Trunk Twist

**Purpose: For trunk, back, and neck.**
- Sitting position with left knee bent and outer side of left leg and ankle contacting the floor. Bring right leg across left and hold in bent knee position with sole of right foot contacting the ground just to the outside of the left thigh.
- Twist torso and turn the head to the right simultaneously, attempting to place both hands to the floor on the right side of the body (keep right leg planted).
- Reverse leg positions and perform movement to left side.

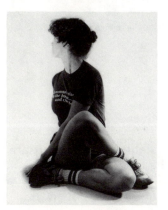

Sitting trunk twist

### Double Arm Hyperextension

**Purpose: For shoulders and chest.**
- Assume standing position.
- Keeping head up and back straight, grasp both hands together behind the back with the elbows extended.
- Raise both arms as far as possible to this position.
- Lower to starting position.

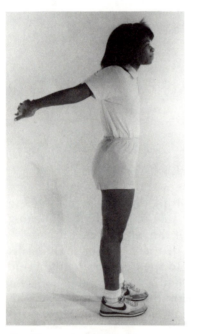

Double arm hyperextension

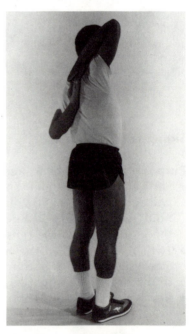

Posterior arm reach

### Posterior Arm Reach

**Purpose: For shoulders, chest, and elbows.**
- Assume standing position.
- Keeping the head up and back straight, place the left arm behind the back, elbow bent and hand facing upward.
- At the same time, place right arm over the right shoulder behind the neck, elbow bent and hand facing downward.

- Attempt to clasp hands.
- Reverse arm positions and execute on opposite side.

**Modified Arm Reach**

- If unable to clasp hands, modify by placing a small towel, ruler, or handkerchief in the hands to help pull arms together.

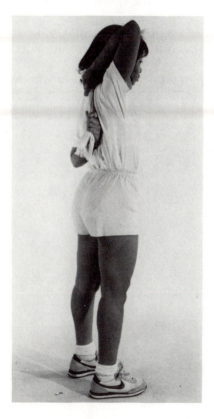

Modified posterior arm reach

**Caution:** The final three movement tasks stress soft tissues of the spine and are advanced exercises that should not be attempted by anyone with structural defects in the upper or lower back regions. If in doubt about readiness to perform them, consult your physician. For those capable of attempting them, perform cautiously!

### Shoulder Stand

**Purpose: For neck and back.**
- Supine position with hands grasping sides of waist, elbows out to the side.
- Bend knees and bring into the chest.
- Attempt to straighten the knees and the spine as the torso is lifted up off the ground.
- Attain as straight a position as possible from shoulders through ankles and support that position with the shoulders and elbows.
- It may be that the torso cannot be lifted entirely off the ground and a fully extended position not be attained. Practice will gradually improve the ability to complete the shoulder stand.

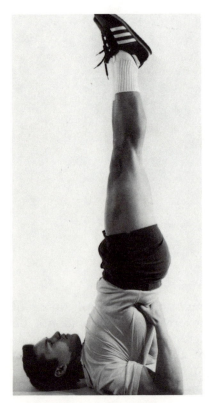

Shoulder stand

### Prone Upper Back Raise (Cobra)

**Purpose: Upper back and trunk.**
- Prone position with the elbows bent and palms of the hands placed on the floor at a point between the chest and the waist.
- Hyperextend the neck and lift the torso off the ground.
- Do not push the body upward with the hands as the elbows are extended! Keep the mid-section in contact with the floor.

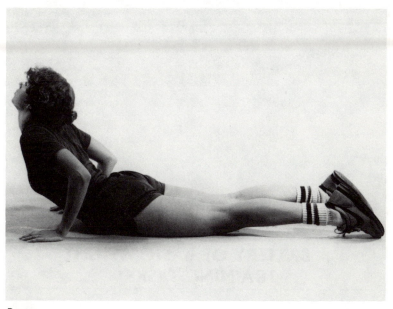

Prone
upper back
raise

### Bent-Knee Spine Stretch

**Purpose: Neck and Back**
- Supine position with arms extended at sides.
- Bend knees and bring into chest.
- Continue to bring legs as far over head as possible in the bent knee position or until you touch the floor above the head with your toes.

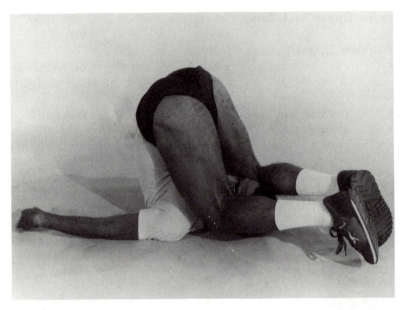

Bent knee
spine
stretch

---

# A BATTERY OF BASIC WEIGHT
# TRAINING TASKS*

---

### General Guidelines and Performance Hints

- Breathe normally while you execute all weight training tasks. Never hold the breath or try to force out air against a sealed windpipe since both are dangerous.
- Execute movements slowly and through full range of motion. Lift rather than swing the weight.

---

*For an extensive range of weight training tasks, let me recommend your consulting: Wayne Webster, *Strength Fitness: Physiological Principles and Training Techniques* (Boston: Allyn and Bacon, Inc., 1982), pp. 119-80.

- Better to start program with too low a resistance and number of reps than with too much.
- In lifting any resistance from the floor, spread the feet, keep the head forward, maintain a straight back, and lower the body to the object by bending at the knees. Then, when lifting, simply straighten the knees.
- Remember — safety first! Free weights should be secured to bars that hold them.

**Arm Curl**

**Purpose: Upper arm, elbow, and wrist.**
- Grasp bar with hands turned inward, arms straight, and elbows close to the sides.
- Keep the back straight as you bring the bar toward the chest by bending the elbows fully.
- Return slowly to the starting position.
- Can be performed with one arm, using a dumbbell.

Arm curl

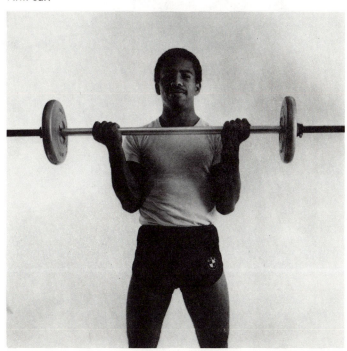

## Military Press

### Purpose: Upper arm, shoulder, elbow, and chest.

- Grasp bar with hands turned outward and bring to the front of the chest at shoulder level.
- Keep the back straight and push the bar slowly overhead by extending the elbows fully.
- Lower to the starting position slowly.
- Can be performed from a bench while lying on the back (bench press) where muscles are capable of handling greater resistance.

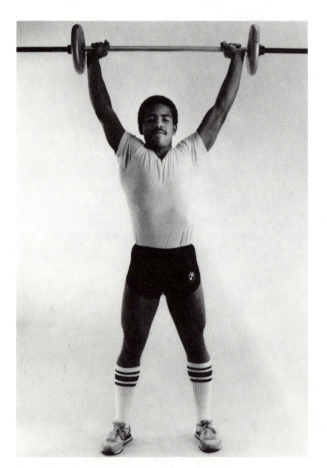

Military press

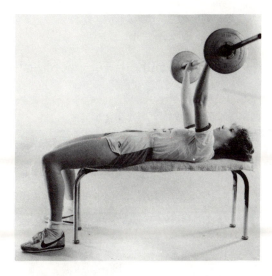

Military press being performed from a bench

## Upright Rowing

**Purpose: Shoulder, upper, outer areas of the back.**
- Grasp bar with the hands turned outward about two inches apart. Place the bar directly in front of the body with the arms straight.
- Pull the bar up by bringing the hands to a position in front of the chest just below the chin, keeping the elbows out to the sides and above the hands.
- Return slowly to the starting position.

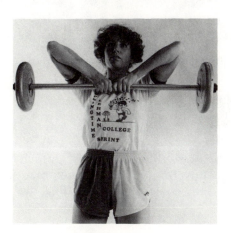

Upright rowing

### Bent Knee Sit-up

**Purpose: Mid-section.**
- Lie on the back with the knees bent and the feet placed flat on the ground.
- Grasp the weight and place below the head.
- Raise the head and chest slowly toward the knees.
- Return slowly to the starting position.
- Feet may be anchored to the ground to keep body stable.
- Can be made more intense by performing on an incline board.

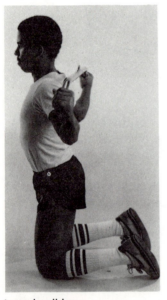 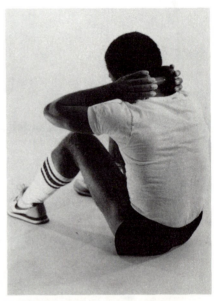

Lateral pulldown        Bent knee sit-up

### Lateral Pulldown

**Purpose: Upper back and arms.**
- Kneel directly under the pull-down bar which is grasped overhead with palms facing outwards and elbows straight.
- Pull the bar down to the upper chest region, bending the elbows slightly.
- Return slowly to the starting position.

### Lateral Arm Raise

**Purpose: Chest.**
- Assume back lying position on the bench, grasping dumbbell with the hands turned inward and elbows straight.
- Raise arms up to the sides and then over the chest, keeping the elbows straight.
- Return slowly to the starting position.

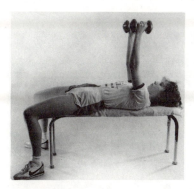

Lateral arm raise

### Knee Extension

**Purpose: Knees and front thigh region.**
- Sit on apparatus with the knees bent and ankles placed under the lifting bar. Place hands on sides of the bench.
- Move the lifting bar upward to a straight knee position, keeping the back straight.
- Return slowly to starting position.

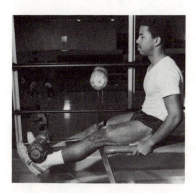

Knee extension

### Knee Flexion (Curl)

**Purpose: Knees and back thigh region.**
- Assume front lying position on the apparatus with knees straight and back of the ankles under the lifting pad.
- Move the lifting bar upward to a bent knee position, trying to keep the hips in contact with the bench.
- Return slowly to the starting position.

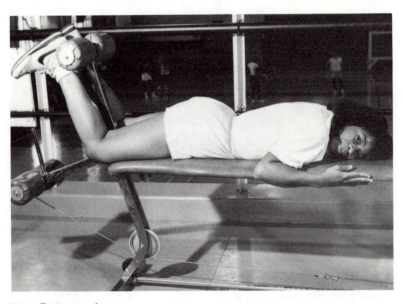

Knee flexion (curl)

### Heel Raise

**Purpose: Ankle and back lower legs.**
- Assume standing position and place bar behind the head at the top of the shoulders.
- Rise up off the heels as far as possible.
- Return slowly to the starting position.
- A greater range of motion can be attained by placing the front portion of the feet on a two to four inch platform.

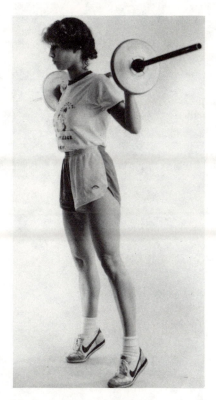

Heel raise

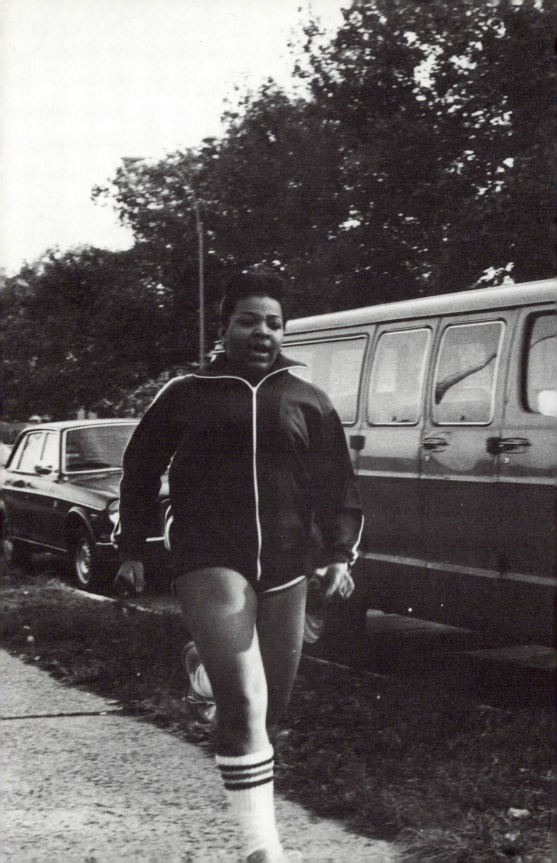

# Chapter Eight

# EXERCISE FOR BODY LEANNESS

*"For we in this generation and in the United States, are the pampered of our planet. . . . We are the fat of the land: never in history, nowhere else in the world have such numbers of human beings eaten so much, exerted themselves so little, and become and remained so fat. We have come suddenly into the land of milk and honey, and we look it. And we suffer because of it."*

Jean Mayer

---

**KEY WORDS**

Kilocalorie
Energy Expenditure
Energy Intake
Energy Balance

Positive Energy Balance
Negative Energy Balance
"Creeping Obesity"
Basal Metabolic Rate

---

## THE CONCEPT OF ENERGY BALANCE

Intricate metabolic processes within body cells involve the production of energy. Basically, fuels furnished from the nutrients we eat are burned in the presence of oxygen. The unit used to measure both energy production within the body and the energy potential of ingested foods is the **kilocalorie (kcal.). A kilocalorie equals the amount of heat (energy) required to raise a kilogram of water one degree centigrade.** The total number of kilocalories you burn or expend over the course of a day (at rest and during the performance of varying activities) is called **energy expenditure** or **caloric output. Energy or caloric intake** is the total number of kcals. contained within the food eaten that day. Like other machines, the body conforms to the principle that energy is neither created nor destroyed but is changed from one form to another. An **energy balance (calorie balance)** is achieved when your energy potential from daily food ingestion equals the total energy you expend that day. **(Energy intake = energy expenditure.)** However, if your daily caloric intake exceeds expenditure, the excess energy in the form of food that remains is converted into fuel stored within the body's fat storage tanks. This is referred to as a positive **energy balance** and, if persistent, would eventually manifest itself in fat accumulation. **(3,500 extra kcal. = approximately one pound of fat.)**

Most of us quite naturally attribute a positive energy balance to overnutrition, that is, overeating resulting from an excessive appetite. We envision the "overeater" as a person with an insatiable desire for food, gorging his or her mouth during meals and constantly raiding the pantry or refrigerator between meals. While this picture sometimes may be justified, an abnormally low daily energy expenditure can also be the culprit, responsible for the production of a positive energy balance. Indeed, there are many of us who do not fit the classic image of the typical foodaholic, yet are guilty of overnourishment because of extremely inactive life-styles and abnormally low caloric outputs.

Have you ever had a sendentary person rationalize that if he were more physically active each day, his appetite would be stimulated, resulting in the consumption of even larger quantities of food! In reality, the very opposite is true. Your appetite will be more excessive when you are physically inactive; and when energy expenditure is made to increase to moderate levels, your desire for food will be more controllable.

It is truly unfortunate that obese people tend to respond

The Obesity Cycle

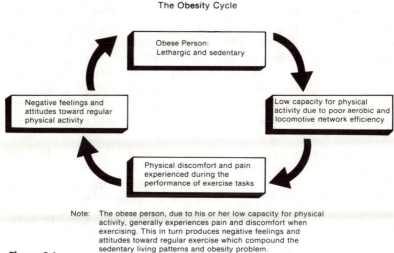

Note: The obese person, due to his or her low capacity for physical activity, generally experiences pain and discomfort when exercising. This in turn produces negative feelings and attitudes toward regular exercise which compound the sedentary living patterns and obesity problem.

**Figure 8.1**

quite negatively to most daily situations that involve increased energy production. When movement tasks are performed, they are most often accomplished with lethargy and too little exuberance, thus detracting from their potential caloric expenditure. A cycle tends to develop whereby the condition of obesity reinforces physical inactivity which further intensifies the condition as well as reducing the potential for other aspects of physical fitness (Figure 8.1).

To reiterate a significant point related in Chapter 3, underexercise or extreme inactivity, like excessive appetite, is quite often symptomatic of some other personal problem. That is to say, it is an overt expression or sign of one or more complex physiological, psychological, or sociocultural conflicts, thus making it most difficult to ameliorate with any degree of success.

## "CREEPING OBESITY"

Let us consider briefly the modern-day condition labeled **"creeping obesity."** This state is experienced by those of you who, while not having a previous obesity problem, begin to put on extra pounds slowly after you reach adult life. In fact, we can define "creeping obesity" as **the gradual accretion of adipose that commences during the early adult (post-college) years.** Generally, the victim of it need not have an excessive number of fat cells. However, those that do exist become much enlarged. The availability of attractive high calorie foods, social drinking, modern modes of transportation, use of appliances, sedentary occupations, and the popularity of inactive recreational pursuits can only contribute to the increase in energy intake and decline in energy expenditure among those who reach early adulthood. Compounding the situation is the fact that a natural reduction in the **basal metabolic rate** (energy expenditure at rest) occurs at this time and continues to drop gradually with each passing year. **Thus, creeping obesity is a threat to every one of you once you reach your twenties.**

## OBESITY ELIMINATION — "THE BIG RIP-OFF"

Most Americans seem only too willing to pay any price for a quick, simple, comfortable method of eliminating their excess body fat once and for all. At first glance, it might appear that there are a number of programs and products on the market today that will accomplish this, but the fact of the matter is that a simple, easy cure for obesity remains to be discovered. While some remedies do bring about temporary weight reductions, most are not only completely ineffective but are hazardous to health. You should be skeptical of crash diets recommended in popular diet books, appetite suppressant drugs, and the host of miracle foods, reducing cocktails, exercise gadgets, vibrating machinery, inflatable limb belts, etc. that come with money-back guarantees. Unfortunately, our federal control agencies (the Federal Trade Commission and the Food and Drug Administration) fail to effectively regulate the sale of fraudulent weight reducing schemes. Evidence for beneficial claims by these charlatan advertisers is not required prior to public sale of their products. They also protect themselves with the strategic loca-

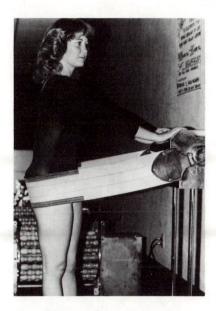

Beware of gadgets that are purported to be an easy cure for obesity.

tion of "fine print" that calls for a routine of difficult procedures to be utilized in conjunction with their product.

Of the 29,000 recorded diet plans in the United States, few are safe and most provide temporary benefits at the most. There are several requisites for an effective, healthy, weight-reduction plan. The drop in the dieter's daily caloric intake depends on how abusive an overeater he is. Generally speaking, the daily curtailment of food intake should be within a range of 200 to less than 1,000 kilocalories unless more is prescribed by a physician. The food that is consumed should be well-proportioned among the basic four groups (dairy, meat, fish, or poultry; whole grains and bread; and fruit and vegetables) and should be accompanied by limitations in the consumption of food products that contain high levels of refined sugars, saturated fats, and salt.

On the other hand, I would question any crash or starvation diet that calls for excessive reduction in daily caloric intake (over 1,000 kcal.) and/or the elimination of a specific food category such as carbohydrates, despite their potential for quick weight reduction. Such a diet will fail to provide adequately for your daily nutritional needs. Excessive fasting (starvation) could also lead to a lowered resistance to infection, anemia, a higher

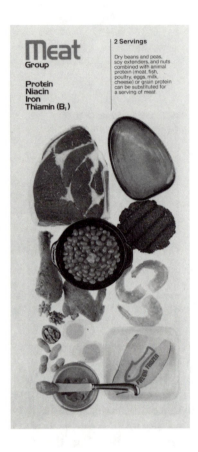

**Meat** Group

Protein
Niacin
Iron
Thiamin (B₁)

2 Servings

Dry beans and peas,
soy extenders, and nuts
combined with animal
protein (meat, fish,
poultry, eggs, milk,
cheese) or grain protein
can be substituted for
a serving of meat

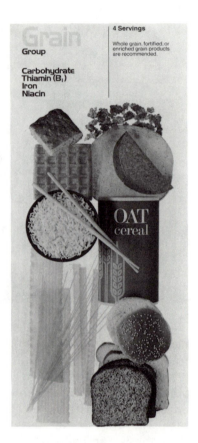

**Grain** Group

Carbohydrate
Thiamin (B₁)
Iron
Niacin

4 Servings

Whole grain, fortified, or
enriched grain products
are recommended.

OAT cereal

than normal blood uric acid level, and excessive water loss. The continual, painful sensation of hunger which invariably accompanies every starvation diet can provoke psychoemotional difficulties including extreme nervousness, tension, anxiety, sleeplessness, and dizziness. Yet, the most valid criticism of a crash diet is its lack of permanency! Because the diet plan is so difficult, if not impossible to maintain, it is quickly abandoned. Once discontinued with regular eating patterns resumed, any weight that was so rapidly discarded with so much suffering is gradually regained. Maybe this is why some people refer to starvation dieting as the "rhythm method of girth control."

There is an extensive list of over-the-counter appetite suppressant drugs. Most have an amphetamine base and are, in reality, legalized "pep pills" which activate the human nervous system. Initially they might curb your desire for food, but since they cause hyperactivity and nervous arousal, you will find great difficulty in relaxing your body and in sleeping at night. Amphetamine is classified as a tolerance drug, which means that the effects of the drug become gradually dissipated with continued use of it. Dosage must be progressively increased to provide the same effects, and such pills are expensive. Thus, in

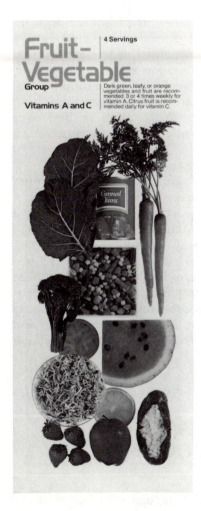

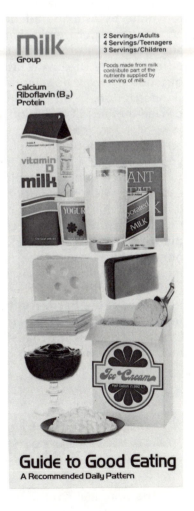

terms of economy, health, and permanency, the diet pill, as an effective means of weight reduction, fails.

Many of us remain confused about the values of dehydration techniques in weight control. Steam and sauna baths, wearing a rubberized suit, or any other procedure that causes profuse sweating might very well produce feelings of satisfaction and comfort. But for permanent weight reduction, they are absolutely worthless, since the decrease in body pounds results solely from water loss and not from energy expenditure. Internal body fluid is essential for homeostasis. Thus, any individual who sweats excessively, whether intended or not, should rehydrate by drinking adequate amounts of liquid. Once ingested, the water weight that was lost will be regained. Finally, any devices that supposedly remove unsightly fat deposits from different body sites with little effort are especially subject to question. There is no scientific evidence as yet to support local slenderization. In other words, except for surgery, there is no proved method of taking off fat from one particular body area as opposed to another. Indeed, when it does occur through an effective technique, the reduction of fat will come from areas of your body where it is most highly concentrated.

In conclusion, we should recognize the fact that the more extreme the degree of obesity, the less hopeful the prognosis. It is indeed much more difficult to control a complex weight problem (evidenced from childhood and continuing through the following stages of life) than if you fall prey to creeping obesity. Recall that, once created, fat cells which have tremendous growth potential can never be destroyed. Thus, there is a very real distinction between obesity control and elimination. **Accept the harsh reality that the struggle against obesity for most of us, especially those in their young adult years and beyond, is endless and that efforts to either control or prevent it must never cease!**

## THE ROLE OF EXERCISE IN THE CONTROL OF OBESITY

The potential contribution that regular exercise can make

to effective obesity control and prevention should be understood by the masses to a much greater extent than it is. The movements of physical activity, you should recall, result from the combustion of fuels, mainly within skeletal muscles (Chapter 3). Thus, when we activate our large muscles, our potential for energy expenditure zooms upward. Consider that an average adult will burn approximately 100 kcals. for every mile he or she walks or jogs. Even jogging at a rather moderate rate of five miles per hour (or one mile in 12 minutes), you will have expended about 35 more kcals. in 12 minutes than would be produced during a full hour of rest. Combining regular exercise and food intake curtailment can easily lead to a **negative energy balance — that is, the expenditure of more kcals. each day than one ingests. Authorities in nutrition, health, and medicine seem to agree that a negative energy balance provides the best hope available for healthy and permanently effective obesity regulation.** It is neither necessary nor desirable to create an excessively large difference in the daily energy intake and expenditure through either exhaustive exercise or severe reduction in food intake that produces hunger.

A mere deficit of 500 calories, which is well within the reach of most people, could lead to a potential loss of one pound per week (500 kcals. × 7 = 3,500 kcal. = 1 lb. fat). Your diet should remain balanced with approximately 15 percent protein, no more than 30 percent fat, and 55 percent carbohydrate. It is best also to spread food ingestion over the course of three or more meals a day to aid in digestion and to curtail the use of highly refined sugars and high calorie foods.

The incorporation of exercise in your obesity control or prevention program is potentially more effective than calorie restriction alone. Weight loss through the latter method alone can occur via the loss of muscle protein, which is not a desirable outcome. Systematic exercise, on the other hand, produces a combination of shrinkage in body fat and the growth of dense muscle-joint tissues. As a matter of fact, this can sometimes result in the maintenance or an increase in your total body weight concomitant with a significant reduction in body fat.

Appropriate caloric costs of several popular physical activities discussed in previous chapters are reported in Table 8.1. (Exact caloric expenditure depends on environmental conditions, degree of intensity with which the task is executed, total body weight, and other variables.)

## Table 8.1

## Approximate Energy Expenditures in Popular Physical Activities Compared to Sitting*

| | Energy Burned Per Half Hour (30 min.) according to Body Weight in Pounds | | | | |
| --- | --- | --- | --- | --- | --- |
| | 90 | 125 | 152 | 205 | 240 |
| Sitting | 22 | 30 | 37 | 49 | 57 |
| Walking | | | | | |
| 2.0 MPH | 63 | 87 | 105 | 144 | 168 |
| 4.4 MPH | 120 | 165 | 201 | 270 | 318 |
| Jogging | | | | | |
| 5.5 MPH | 192 | 270 | 324 | 438 | 513 |
| 7.0 MPH | 252 | 351 | 423 | 570 | 669 |
| Cycling | | | | | |
| 5.5 MPH | 90 | 127 | 153 | 204 | 240 |
| 13.0 MPH | 192 | 267 | 324 | 438 | 513 |
| Rope Skipping | 236 | 328 | 399 | 538 | 630 |
| Swimming (Front Crawl) | | | | | |
| 25 yds/min. | 108 | 150 | 183 | 256 | 288 |
| 50 yds/min. | 192 | 267 | 321 | 435 | 510 |
| Calisthenics and Stretching | 90 | 126 | 153 | 204 | 240 |
| Lifetime Sports | | | | | |
| Golf | 72 | 102 | 123 | 169 | 190 |
| Racquetball | 177 | 243 | 297 | 396 | 468 |
| Tennis | 126 | 174 | 210 | 282 | 330 |
| Downhill Skiing | 174 | 243 | 294 | 393 | 462 |
| Cross Country Skiing | 236 | 328 | 396 | 538 | 630 |
| Dancing | | | | | |
| Moderate Social | 79 | 105 | 126 | 171 | 201 |
| Vigorous Social | 102 | 141 | 176 | 231 | 273 |
| Square Dancing | 123 | 171 | 207 | 279 | 327 |

*Often neglected is the fact that your energy expenditure can remain elevated for several hours following exercise as the body recovers from it!

## Approximate Energy Expenditures of Various Physical Activities Compared with Sitting*

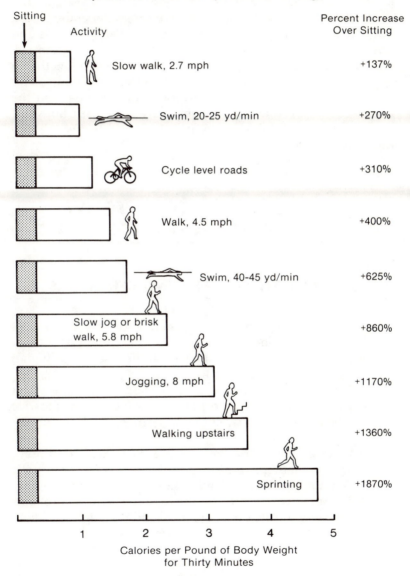

| Sitting | Activity | Percent Increase Over Sitting |
|---|---|---|
| | Slow walk, 2.7 mph | +137% |
| | Swim, 20-25 yd/min | +270% |
| | Cycle level roads | +310% |
| | Walk, 4.5 mph | +400% |
| | Swim, 40-45 yd/min | +625% |
| | Slow jog or brisk walk, 5.8 mph | +860% |
| | Jogging, 8 mph | +1170% |
| | Walking upstairs | +1360% |
| | Sprinting | +1870% |

Calories per Pound of Body Weight
for Thirty Minutes

*Johnson, Perry, et al. Sport, Exercise and You. New York:
Holt, Rinehart and Winston, 1975, p. 289.

**Figure 8.2**

A combination of moderate exercise and food curtailment is not an artificial or synthetic method of losing weight. The success of this type of obesity control program depends, in part, upon your knowledge of caloric values of varying foods and physical activities. Faithful adherence to such a program will definitely be more demanding and difficult to swallow than a reducing pill, but it will produce lasting effects. Of course, it is essential that you enjoy both the foods that you eat and the exercise you perform. Outlined below are some basic hints that should prove helpful to your creating an effective obesity regulation program of this type.

# HELPFUL HINTS FOR EFFECTIVE OBESITY REGULATION

## MODIFICATION OF EATING BEHAVIORS

- Learn to judge the caloric potential of varying portions and kinds of food.
- Attempt to substitute lower calorie foods for higher calorie ones (see Table 8.2).
- Either eliminate or reduce the portions of fattening foods you tend to consume (e.g., nuts, gravies, potato chips, ice cream, candy, soda, cookies, pastries, alcoholic beverages, etc.).
- Beware of fried foods — choose lower kcal. food preparation methods.
- Don't buy and keep high kcal. foods around the house.
- Try not to skip meals — in the long run, you will probably eat more during one large meal and find digestion more difficult than if you consume several smaller meals.
- Eat slowly — try more conversation during eating and make meals more social.
- At each meal, stop eating before you are completely full.
- An hour to half hour before a meal, consume a small carbohydrate snack (e.g., fruit or cereal) if you desire to curb a ravenous appetite.

**Table 8.2**

**Examples of Reducing Calories through Food Substitution**

| Food | Kcal. | Substitute | Kcal. | Kcal. Saved |
|---|---|---|---|---|
| 8 oz. milk | 165 | Skim milk | 80 | 85 |
| 8 oz. prune juice | 170 | Tomato juice | 50 | 120 |
| 8 oz. soda | 105 | Water | 0 | 105 |
| 8 oz. malted milk shake | 500 | Lemonade | 100 | 400 |
| 2 scrambled eggs | 220 | 2 boiled eggs | 160 | 60 |
| Buttered toast | 170 | Jelly on toast | 80 | 90 |
| Chocolate cake, 2″ piece | 425 | Plain cake, 2″ piece | 115 | 310 |
| Apple pie, piece | 345 | Tangerine or ½ cantaloupe | 40 | 305 |
| 2 oz. hamburger | 240 | 3 oz. chicken roast | 160 | 80 |
| 3 oz. pork chop | 340 | 3 oz. veal chop | 185 | 150 |
| 10 potato chips | 115 | Grapes, 1 cup | 65 | 35 |
| French fried potatoes, 1 cup | 480 | 1 potato, baked | 100 | 380 |

# MODIFICATION OF PHYSICAL ACTIVITY BEHAVIORS

- Try to become more "kcal. burning" conscious. Replace everyday sedentary habits with more physically active ones (walk instead of using the car, bus, or subway; substitute the staircase for the elevator; take the bicycle to the store, etc.).
- Perform some form of recreational exercise every day. It will be psychologically rewarding as well as physiologically beneficial.
- Recreational exercise need not be exhaustive.
- Try to develop interest in a variety of physical activities that you can perform on a regular basis.
- When hungry, exercise! It will curb rather than increase appetite.

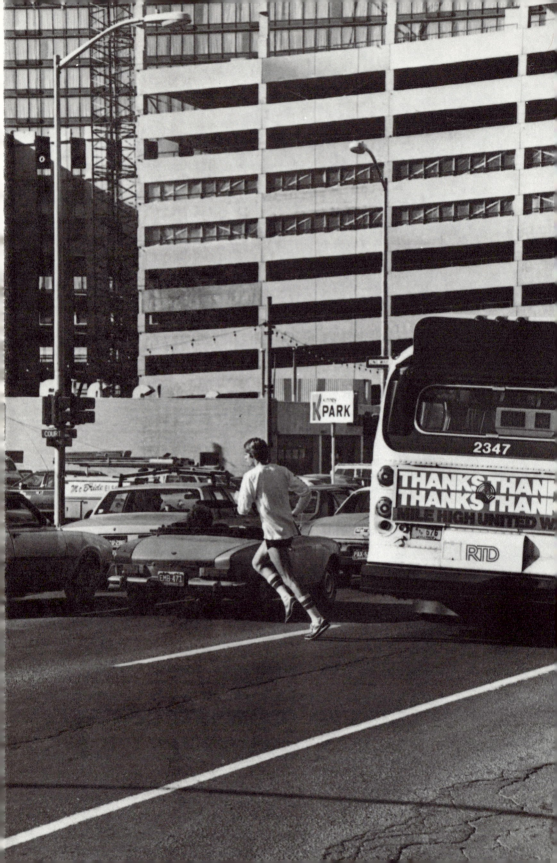

# Chapter Nine

# EXERCISE PRECAUTIONS AND RECOMMENDATIONS FOR EFFECTIVE BODY CARE

*"The head cannot say to the feet, I have no need of thee! . . . God has so adjusted the body that there may be no discord. If one member suffers all suffer together, if one member is honored all rejoice together."*

*St. Paul (First Corinthians)*

---

**KEY WORDS**

Acclimatization
Hypothermia
Muscle Cramp

Heat Stroke
"Overexercise"

---

# POOR AIR QUALITY

A word of caution is warranted for urban dwellers and any others of you who might be inclined to exercise in the vicinity of heavy auto traffic, factories, incinerators, airports, or other environs where the air is likely to be saturated with pollutants that are dangerous to health. The upper portion of your air intake track does have a natural filter system that can inhibit the passage of large foreign materials into the lungs, but small, harmful solids and gases are not intercepted. Remember that larger than normal volumes of air are inspired during exercise, and if impure in content could cause nausea, headache, or perhaps even some internal tissue damage.

When air quality in your residential area is poor, indoor, rather than outdoor, exercise might be more appropriate for you. And, obviously, when engaging in outdoor physical activities, try to seek localities such as parks, grassy fields, meadows, and open surroundings with an abundance of nearby plant life where the air is more clear, rather than those in close proximity to sources of pollution.

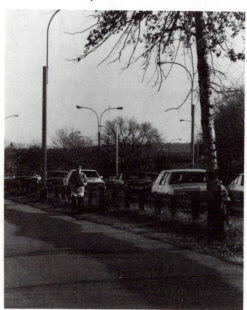

Try to avoid exercising in environments that are unhealthy and potentially dangerous in terms of accidents.

# EXERCISE IN EXTREMELY WARM AND COLD WEATHER CONDITIONS

Your body is programmed for **acclimatization, that is, the maintenance of normal internal body temperature when you are exposed to either extremely warm or cold weather conditions.** It is prudent to curtail dosage during initial exercise bouts in either case, because full adjustment occurs with gradual exposure (somewhere between two to four days) to the prevailing type of weather extreme. You should also recognize that there is always the possibility of a breakdown in your temperature control mechanisms which can pose serious complications!

Core body temperature can be magnified as much as twenty times resting level during periods of stressful muscular use. It is our blood that actually transfers this internal heat from the muscles to the skin where it is given off to the outside air. An extensively warm environment is not conducive to this heat

Internal tissue fluid is lost via sweating and increased respiration. It is sound practice to replace it by drinking liquids before, during, and after exercise; whether thirsty or not. It is also wise to try to cool the body down by water dousing when exercising in extreme heat.

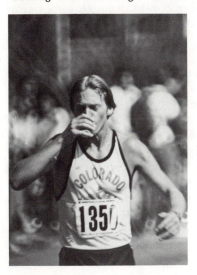
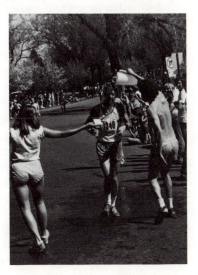

exchange. Excessive humidity compounds the difficulty in that we rely on the air's absorption of heat from our skin surface to keep the core temperature from climbing. Although perspiration is likely to occur, the sweat you produce fails to evaporate readily, causing less body heat to be transferred. A large volume of tissue fluid (water and dissolved minerals) is invariably taken from the blood as you sweat profusely which, in turn, can precipitate a fluid deficiency in your body, unless replaced as it is lost.

**The reduction of body fluids or increase in body temperature (or a combination of both, which is usually the case) can create states of being that are uncomfortable, incapacitating, and even life threatening.** It would be wise for all who exercise, especially those of you who do so exclusively in warm environments, to learn the symptoms, treatment, and preventive measures for the common heat-related body conditions presented in Table 9.1. Keep in mind also that as each of us gets on in years, the body's tolerance of heat dwindles progressively. Physical activities performed in hot weather conditions require your heart to work harder, as evidenced by a higher heart rate response to exercise, than it does under more comfortably cool ones. Thus, people above their middle-aged years and/or those of you below moderate levels of fitness might do well to alter exercise efforts when warm weather conditions prevail.

Exposure to severe winter-like conditions including below freezing temperatures, icy winds, and precipitation can also cause havoc for the exerciser. They could result in an excessive decline in body temperature *(hypothermia)* as well as producing frostbite (the crystallization and eventual destruction of skin and underlying tissues), mainly to limbs and exposed portions of the face. Cold air entering the air intake track coats the chest and neck linings, and this results in a reduction in the volume of blood flowing from this region to the arteries located within the walls of the heart. The lowered level of circulation means less oxygen availability to the tissues that comprise these walls and, thus, contributes to their potential damage. Evidently, one should proceed with exercise in the cold environment only when absolutely certain the heart is both healthy and functionally fit. Even if you are fit, be sure to increase warm-up time and start out in exercise slowly with a more gradual intensification of energy output than normal. Be cognizant of the fact

## Table 9.1

## Disabling Conditions Associated with Exercise and Excessive Body Heat

| Condition | Tell Tale Signs | Treatment |
|---|---|---|
| **Muscle Cramping**<br><br>Debilitating but not too serious condition. Muscle goes into state of involuntary contraction. | • Part or whole muscle tightens.<br>• Limb incapacitation.<br>• Pain.<br>• Calf muscle (posterior lower leg) most common site. | • Stop activity.<br>• Rest.<br>• Replace fluids.<br>• Add table salt to foods. |
| **Heat Exhaustion**<br><br>Temporary, incapacitating illness that most often occurs with initial exposure to warm weather and/or penetrating sun rays. | • Headache.<br>• Nausea.<br>• Weakness.<br>• Clammy Skin. | • Get out of sun.<br>• Rest.<br>• Cool shower.<br>• Cool fluids (if not nauseous). |
| **Heat Stroke**<br><br>Complicated, somewhat mysterious state in which heat regulatory mechanisms fail. Excessive internal temperature can cause shock and death. | • High fever (102-106°).<br>• Pulse - rapid, faint.<br>• Skin - hot, dry, and red.<br>• Loss of awareness.<br>• Shock.<br>• Unconsciousness. | • Curtail exercise immediately.<br>• Lower internal temperature immediately - douse with any cold liquid available.<br>• Apply ice or cold towels.<br>• Send for emergency medical help. |

## Preventive Measures for the Above Conditions

• Wear a cap to protect head from sun rays.
• Light weight and perforated clothing with adequate limb exposure promotes the dissipation of heat from the skin surfaces. Lighter colors are preferred, since they reflect rather than absorb sun rays.

*(continued)*

**Table 9.1** *(continued)*

- Avoid rubberized suits and any clothing or equipment that blocks the passage of heat from the skin to the air. They do not promote permanent weight reduction as many believe and can be quite hazardous in that they cause the elevation of internal body temperature.
- Drink fluids (water, fruit juices, and/or commercial athletic drinks) before, during, and following exercise bouts that produce excessive sweating. Do so whether thirsty or not!
- Add salted foods to the diet and/or sprinkle extra table salt on foods in anticipation of and following heavy sweating. Consumption of salt tablets is not advocated! Excessive salt tends to irritate the stomach lining and has also been implicated as a risk factor in high blood pressure.
- On extremely warm humid days: (1) curtail exercise efforts, (2) confine them to a water environment (where overheating will not occur) and/or exercise during the early or later portions of the day when heat is less intense.

---

**Table 9.2**

## Precautionary Measures when Exercising in Extremely Cold Weather Conditions

- Use thermal under and outerwear.
- Wear gloves, face mask, and hat.
- Wear parka or other clothing made with goose down material which is highly insulating.
- Wear several layers of light clothing — these are more protective and less cumbersome than one heavy, bulky layer and can be discarded more readily if no longer needed.
- Do not overdress when temperature and winds are not that severe. Too much clothing could cause wet undergarments from perspiration, and this can be both uncomfortable and chill producing.
- Go indoors periodically from the cold for a warm drink, to thaw limbs, and to dry outer garments if wet.
- Wear water resistant outer garments when exposed to snow or rain in addition to cold. Hypothermia tends to occur more rapidly when clothing is wet (even in temperatures above freezing). Wet clothing provides little insulation and actually accelerates the loss of internal body heat.

that the colder your locomotive and service networks, the lower their potential level of operational effectiveness!

Those of you who desire it and are capable of performing cold weather physical activity (jogging, ice skating, skiing, ice boating, snow shoveling, etc.) can offset the effects of your exposure to frigid temperatures and winds by taking the precautionary actions presented in Table 9.2.

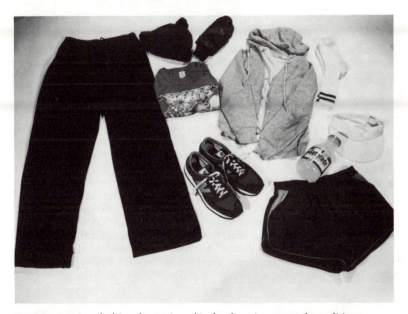

Proper exercise clothing for various kinds of environmental conditions.

## NUTRITION CONSIDERATIONS

It was stated previously (Chapter 2) that your body automatically converts the table foods you eat into the metabolic substances required for the operation, repair, and growth of all your body tissues. The production of quality exercise fuels is assured by the everyday consumption of proper amounts of nourishing foods. **The consensus of nutrition experts is that everyone who exercises (from the athlete engaged in vigorous**

## Table 9.3

## Basic Nutrition Guidelines for the Exerciser

- Daily food intake should be balanced. A well-rounded diet would include approximately:
    15% Protein
    30% Fat (20% unsaturated, 10% saturated)
    55% Carbohydrate
- Total daily fuel intake (in kilocalories) should be equivalent to the energy expended by the body.
- Decrease the consumption of saturated fat (red meats and animal fat products such as eggs, whole milk, butter, cheeses, cream, etc.). These fats are associated with the production of materials that can gather on the inner linings of blood vessels within the heart and brain. The vessels narrow progressively and the circulation of blood through these vital organs is impeded. This process reduces their level of functioning and eventually can cause fatal damage to them.
- Consume more poly-unsaturated and mono-saturated fat products such as vegetable, olive, and sunflower oils and margarine.
- Limit the consumption of refined white sugar and foods prepared with it (pastry, cookies, doughnuts, ice cream, candy, and soda). They are high in caloric content and low in nutritional value.
- Consume more poultry, veal, fish, legumes (beans, peas, and lentils) and "complex carbohydrates" such as fresh vegetables, fruits, and whole grains. Their caloric content is not excessive while their nutritive value is high.

**training for competition to the person in pursuit of optimal fitness) can provide quite adequately for daily nutritional needs via a normal, well-balanced diet.** Give due consideration, therefore, to the basic nutrition recommendations outlined in Table 9.3. Generally, if these guidelines are followed, you need not spend money on vitamin, mineral, or protein supplements to your diet. In actuality, they fail to promote significant nutritional benefits, despite the advertised claims of their manufacturers to do so.

Exceptions to the principle of "proper diet, no additives," are the possible advantages that might be derived from the consumption of extra carbohydrate over a period of one to three days prior to the performance of an excessively high energy expenditure exercise bout. Many today seem to derive a great deal of satisfaction from the challenge of prolonged physical activities. Here, the extra carbohydrate consumption could very well add somewhat to the glucose content within the body, which, in turn, would take working muscles a longer period of time to deplete during the extensive exercise performance.

Eating "sweets" such as candy bars before exercise, although quite commonly done, is, on the other hand, counterproductive to the performance of a physical activity. Those of you who do so, erroneously contend that the carbohydrate ingested will give you "quick" energy. On the contrary, the sugar that enters the blood tends to stimulate the production of insulin, a hormone that reduces the muscle's ability to burn fatty acids. Thus, working muscles must rely to a greater degree on glucose as their fuel for energy production. This places greater demands on the glucose reserves located within the blood, muscles, and liver which, in turn, are more rapidly exhausted.

Critical mineral substances such as potassium and sodium can also be depleted as a result of frequent exercise, more so if large amounts of tissue fluids are lost by way of sweating. Their absence from the body can quicken fatigue as well as muscle weakness, resulting ultimately in a reduced level of exercise performance. You could offset the possible draining of these valuable minerals by adding a little more table salt to your foods (Table 9.1) and by increasing your consumption of fresh fruits and citrus juices which are high in potassium content (bananas and orange juice especially).

# RELAXATION AND SLEEP

Proper rest and sleep, like nourishing foods, are body revitalizers. They provide opportunities between exercise workouts for the locomotive and service tissues to repair and recharge themselves and are, therefore, critical to your overall body care and health maintenance. Much speculation exists concerning sleep requirements. Suffice it to say that suitable daily sleep is an individual matter — some of you requiring as little as four hours and others as much as ten hours of it. Either too much or too little sleep can affect personality and human performance, including that of physical activities. Deviation from normal sleep patterns and the inability to relax can be indicators of overstress to the body from too much exercise or insufficient recovery from it. Under such circumstances, you would tend to wear yourself out and lower your state of physical health and fitness rather than improve it.

All of you who do exercise on a regular basis, particularly those engaged in vigorous conditioning regimens, might benefit greatly (both physiologically and psychologically) from a period or two of daily relaxation. True relaxation brings about a significantly lower degree of activation within all body organs including those within regulatory, locomotive, and service networks. The reduced level of metabolic functioning resulting from this is believed to be quite refreshing and restorative in terms of the recovery (of both the individual organs and the total body) from varying kinds of stress. And, those of you who

Two ways to relax your body.

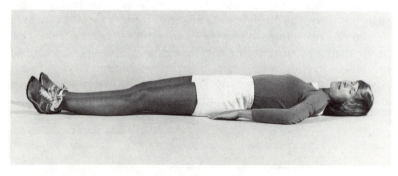

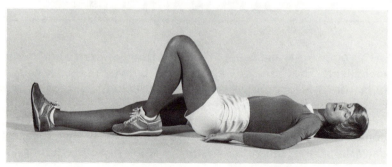

have insomnia, nervousness, anxiety, or other exercise recovery problems might alleviate them at least to some degree through the practice of the simplified relaxation guidelines that are presented in Table 9.4.

## Table 9.4

## Simplified Relaxation Procedures

- Assume comfortable position (lying on the back or a semi-reclining one with feet supported in elevated position) in quiet area.
- Relax and close the eyes.
- Breathe deeply and slowly for about two minutes, focusing your mind completely on your breathing and feelings of internal warmness.
- Immobilize and relax your entire network of muscles and joints completely. It might help to deactivate gradually by beginning at your feet and progressing upward toward the face. Simply "let go" of all internal feelings within each locomotive area.
- After immobilizing your facial muscles, keep your brain inactivated by continuing to focus your thoughts on your breathing.
- You should neither encourage thoughts of any kind, nor should you force them from your mind should they enter it.
- Remain in this position for 15-20 minutes.
- Try to inactivate yourself in this manner at least once a day.

# PROFESSIONAL SERVICES FOR EXERCISE-RELATED DISABILITIES

One must never lose sight of the fact that exercise is a form of stress to the body. While subjection to suitable levels of it can enhance your physical health and fitness, a number of disabling conditions can be precipitated via the performance of different physical activities. Accidental injury, the constant practice of faulty movement patterns, use of improper equipment and facilities, and "overexercise" can either lead to problems or compound existing ones. It is not unusual, therefore, for damage and failure within locomotive, service, and other body parts to occur periodically among a great number of exercise enthusiasts.

**Pain is your body's chief trouble indicator.** Unusual and/or lingering and recurrent pain during or following exercise is cause for concern. Discoloration, deformity, swelling, and abnormal sounds also reflect locomotive parts that are defective and in need of repair. When such symptoms are severe, persistent, and reappear often, you should definitely consult a professional specialist trained to diagnose and treat the problem that exists.

Major remedies for exercise-related disabilities and infirmities include surgery, medication, corrective therapy, use of special equipment, and, at times, simply rest. It would be foolish and dangerous for you to ignore any abnormal symptoms and to continue with your exercise efforts with the hope that they might alleviate the condition. More often than not, exercise will intensify the movement-related disability or illness rather than cure it. Table 9.5 provides a simple reference chart that denotes the professional to consult when physical shortcomings are evidenced.

**Table 9.5**

**Professionals Specializing in Services for
Exercise-Related Disabilities**

| Machine Part Affected | Specialist |
| --- | --- |
| General illnesses and disabilities | General Physician and Internist |
| Heart and other service organs | Cardiologist — Internist |
| Feet | Podiatrist — Orthopedist |
| Muscles, bones, joints | Orthopedist |
| Skin | Dermatologist |

# "OVEREXERCISE"

Some of us apply the popular philosophy, "If something is good for us, twice as much is better!" to our exercise endeavors. **Pushing yourself beyond your limits for tolerating the demands of physical activity or failing to provide sufficient opportunity for body recuperation from them could produce a variety of troublesome outcomes as indicated in Table 9.6.** If you experience any of these symptoms, you are probably overdoing it with your exercise performance. Curtail your dosage immediately (intensity, duration, and/or frequency), and see if the symptoms disappear. If they do not, it might be wise to seek medical help.

**Table 9.6**

**Symptoms of "Overexercise"**

- Lag or drop in exercise performance. In sports, athletic skills capacity becomes markedly reduced.
- Insomnia, difficulty in getting to sleep, or inability to fall back to sleep after awakening during the night.
- Persistent pain, stiffness, soreness, or heaviness in muscles and joints.
- Frequent and lingering illness such as colds and sore throats.
- Loss of appetite.
- Excessive thirst.
- Nervousness, anxiety, and inability to relax.
- Personality changes including irritability, loss of patience, and reduced self-confidence.
- Clumsiness.

# PROTECTION OF WEIGHT-BEARING BODY PARTS IN EXERCISE

**Safety should be the ultimate concern of everyone who exercises. The more inherently dangerous the physical activity**

**you perform, the greater need for quality in the protective and injury resistive clothing and equipment you select.** A good athletic bra for a female and supporter for a male, for instance, will provide protection and prevent sagging and stretching in the body parts they cover.

Performing physical activities in the upright position can be quite traumatic to the weight-bearing regions of your body including the feet, ankles, knees, hips, and spine. **Their overall health and protection, believe it or not, begins with proper care of the feet.** While the shock of striking the ground each time with full body weight is borne by the foot, it is immediately transmitted upward to the other weight-bearing joints.

Composed of twenty-six bones and close to twice that number of ligaments and muscles, the human foot is truly a remarkable piece of apparatus (Figure 9.1A). Strong, resilient, well-formed feet provide the key to the stability and resiliency of the rest of the body in bearing the stress of its own weight when moving in the standing position. If abnormalities exist within them (whether inherent or acquired), they will soon begin to adversely affect other supportive joint structures, usually starting at the ankles or knees and continuing upward to the spine. Although sometimes difficult to accept, the fact remains that back problems often emanate from problem feet.

**Sound footwear is the major requisite to effective care and protection of your feet and thus to the prevention of disabilities to them as well as to other related joints.** Purchasing a quality athletic shoe, even if costing a few extra dollars, is a wise investment. Whether selecting a ski boot, running shoe, or tennis sneaker, it should be constructed with high grade materials, designed effectively, and should fit properly. The major features to seek in a sound athletic shoe used for walking and jogging are presented in Figure 9.1B. When buying your athletic footwear, take the time to examine it carefully. Does it have a good, high arch support? Is the sole of the shoe sturdy and thick? Does the outside covering seem strong and resilient? If you can't twist and bend the shoe back and forth and from side to side very easily, it probably has good strength and stability. For comfort, it should have a soft, well-cushioned inner sole. Once purchased, keep your footwear in good repair. In cases where problem feet are known to exist (e.g., flat feet or high arches) inserts can be fitted to most shoes for extra protection

Ankle-Foot Structure and Major
Features of a Quality Jogging Shoe

A. Ankle - Foot Structure

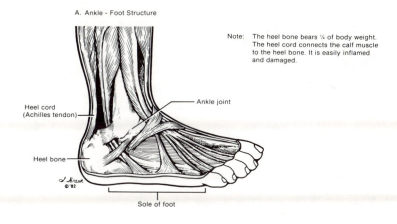

Note:    The heel bone bears ¼ of body weight.
         The heel cord connects the calf muscle
         to the heel bone. It is easily inflamed
         and damaged.

Heel cord
(Achilles tendon)

Ankle joint

Heel bone

Sole of foot

B. Quality Jogging Shoe

Heel counter

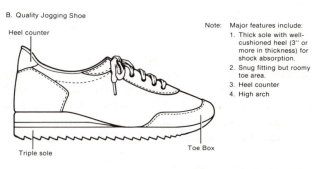

Note:    Major features include:
         1. Thick sole with well-
            cushioned heel (3" or
            more in thickness) for
            shock absorption.
         2. Snug fitting but roomy
            toe area.
         3. Heel counter
         4. High arch

Triple sole

Toe Box

**Figure 9.1**

by a competent podiatrist. The white athletic sock that covers
the foot should be clean and also fit snugly. Abiding by these
simple precautions can help you avoid a variety of potential
**problems — the major ones being blisters, heel-bruises, knee-
aches, shin-splints, strains, sprains, and (Achilles) tendonitis.**

# "TROUBLESHOOTING GUIDE"

A listing of the more common traumatic difficulties and
problems encountered by those who exercise is provided in the

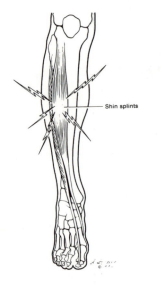

**Figure 9.2**
Shin splints

guide below (Table 9.7). By gaining insight into their causation, hopefully you will be able to take measures to prevent their occurrence. Since many of these troubles cannot always be prevented, the information provided in this "troubleshooting" guide should also assist you in the recognition of the condition and the appropriate action to take should it arise.

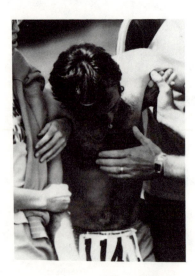

Table 9.7

## Troubleshooting Guide

| Problem | Warning Signals | Potential Causes | Corrective Measures | Preventive Measures |
|---|---|---|---|---|
| **Blisters** (Small friction burns common to toes, feet, ankle, heel, fingers, and palm of hands). | • Redness<br>• Heat<br>• Small fluid filled bubble usually clear but sometimes reddish if blood is present. | • Heat from friction caused by constant rubbing of material against skin areas (e.g., shoes too tight or loose). | • Pad affected area for comfort and to reduce friction.<br>• Clean and disinfect if blister breaks.<br>• See general physician if severe. | • Avoid friction.<br>• Proper sock and shoe fit.<br>• Gloves for hands.<br>• Pad or coat (with vaseline) areas prone to friction. |
| **Bursitis** (Usually shoulder or elbow. | • Pain within joint.<br>• Intensified upon limb movement.<br>• Movement incapacitation. | • Inflammation of bursae sacs within joint (fluid accumulation).<br>• Could be inherent in origin or due to overuse of joint or injury.<br>• Can be chronic. | • Immediate cold application.<br>• Immobility.<br>• Heat following cessation of fluid accumulation.<br>• See orthopedist if symptoms are severe. | • Avoid overuse.<br>• Flexibility exercises. |
| **Chonromalacia** "Runner's Knee" | • Persistent pain under knee cap.<br>• Knee swelling.<br>• Knee stiffness, especially following sleep and other periods of holding knee in same position.<br>• Catching or locking of knee during use. | • Rubbing of bones which articulate at knee.<br>• Precipitated by faulty knees and feet.<br>• Overuse via excessive jogging. | • See orthopedic surgeon. | • Curtail jogging and other exercise performed in upright position.<br>• Shoe inserts. |
| **Dyspnea** (Painful Breathing) | • Severe discomfort and/ or pain experienced when rate and depth of breathing are elevated. | • Ineffective respiratory mechanisms.<br>• Could be due to failure to exercise regularly.<br>• Could be precipitated by defective lungs or air intake track (emphysema or other diseases). | • Participation in systematic aerobic exercise.<br>• See general physician if condition persists. | • Participation in systematic aerobic exercise.<br>• Avoid cigarette smoking. |
| **Heart Defects** | • Chest pain (mild to crushing intensity).<br>• Burning or tingling sensation in neck, jaw, inner arm, upper midsection, or between shoulders.<br>• Sudden indigestion and possible nausea.<br>• Cold sweat<br>• Paleness. | • Faulty blood vessels within heart's muscular walls (blockage, narrowing or bursting). | • Cease exercise immediately.<br>• Assume sitting or semireclining position with legs supported in bentknees position above hips.<br>• Call physician or get to hospital.<br>• Try to remain calm. | • No certain preventive procedures.<br>• Proper food intake, regular exercise, abstaining from cigarettes, stress avoidance, and maintaining leanness might help. |
| **Joint Sprain or Strain** (Most often to ankle) | • Pain.<br>• Swelling.<br>• Discoloration. | • Accidental injury — severe twisting or pushing joint beyond normal type of range of motion causing rupture or tearing of soft tissues and fluid accumulation. | • Immediate application of cold over affected and adjacent areas.<br>• Compression Bandage.<br>• Elevation.<br>• If severe, see general physician or take x-ray. | • Proper athletic footwear.<br>• Regular heel cord stretching. |

*(continued)*

**Table 9.7 (continued)**

| Problem | Warning Signals | Potential Causes | Corrective Measures | Preventive Measures |
|---|---|---|---|---|
| **Low Back Pain** | • Mild to crippling pain in lower back region.<br>• Stiffness.<br>• Abnormal curve in lower as well as upper back ("sway back").<br>• Sagging mid-section often present. | • Range of possible causes.<br>• More serious cases due to defects in spinal column (inherent or acquired).<br>• Often can be attributed to weakness in musculature of back and mid-section as well as lack of flexibility in spine. | **(Severe Conditions)**<br>• Surgery.<br>• Rest (traction)<br><br>**(Milder Conditions)**<br>• Corrective exercises to stretch spine and enhance condition of back and mid-section muscles. | • Regular exercise to keep weight down.<br>• Stretching and muscle endurance exercises for spine and mid-section. |
| **Muscle Strain**<br>"Pulled Muscle"<br>(Common to back thigh area.) | • Sharp, local pain.<br>• Limb immobility.<br>• Slight swelling. | • Tearing of tissues in muscle due to violent stretching.<br>• Often precipitated by strength imbalance of opposing muscle groups (e.g., front thigh muscle motors much stronger than back thigh group).<br>• Over use of muscle motors. | • Immediate cold.<br>• Rest.<br>• Heat following cessation of swelling. | • Flexibility exercises that stretch muscles and tendons.<br>• Strengthen weak muscles. |
| **Muscle Soreness** | • Pain.<br>• Stiffness.<br>• Heaviness.<br>• Loss of mobility. | • Over use of muscle motors. | • Rest.<br>• Heat applications.<br>• Light activation following recovery. | • Proper exercise dosage — avoid overuse.<br>• Gradual progression in exercise dosage when commencing exercise program. |

**Overheating Conditions (see Table 9.1, p. 173)**

| Problem | Warning Signals | Potential Causes | Corrective Measures | Preventive Measures |
|---|---|---|---|---|
| **Shin Splints** | • Pain in front lower leg, especially upon walking or running.<br>• Sensitivity to touch. | • Tearing or inflammation of tendons of muscles or membranes located between lower leg bones. | • Cold application.<br>• Rest. | • Could be chronic.<br>• Avoid or curtail weight-bearing exercise performed in an upright position.<br>• Proper exercise shoe, running on soft surfaces.<br>• Corrective shoe inserts. |
| **Stress Fractures**<br>(Hairline crack in bone) | • Severe pain, especially upon limb movement.<br>• Sensitivity to touch | • Overuse (constant pounding and shock of movement). | • Curtail exercise.<br>• Immobilize.<br>• See general physician or orthopedist | • Proper athletic footwear.<br>• Avoid overuse.<br>• Jogging or running on soft surfaces. |
| **Tendonitis**<br>(Achilles or "Heel cord" tendon most common) | • Pain<br>• Swelling<br>• Sensitivity to touch (tendon area) | • Slight rips in tendon or covering membrane of muscle. | • Cold application.<br>• Rest.<br>• Heat following cessation of swelling. | • Proper athletic footwear.<br>• Heel cord stretching before and after exercise.<br>• Running on soft surfaces. |
| **Traumatic Elbow**<br>("Tennis elbow") | • Elbow pain, especially upon movement.<br>• Swelling.<br>• Movement incapacitation. | • Tears in joint tendons and/or other soft tissues within elbow.<br>• Often precipitated by faulty patterns and overuse of elbow (not only in tennis but in other activities as well). | • Cold application.<br>• Rest.<br>• Compression.<br>• See orthopedist if severe. | • Proper elbow movement.<br>• Avoid overuse.<br>• Flexibility and weight training exercises for elbow might help. |

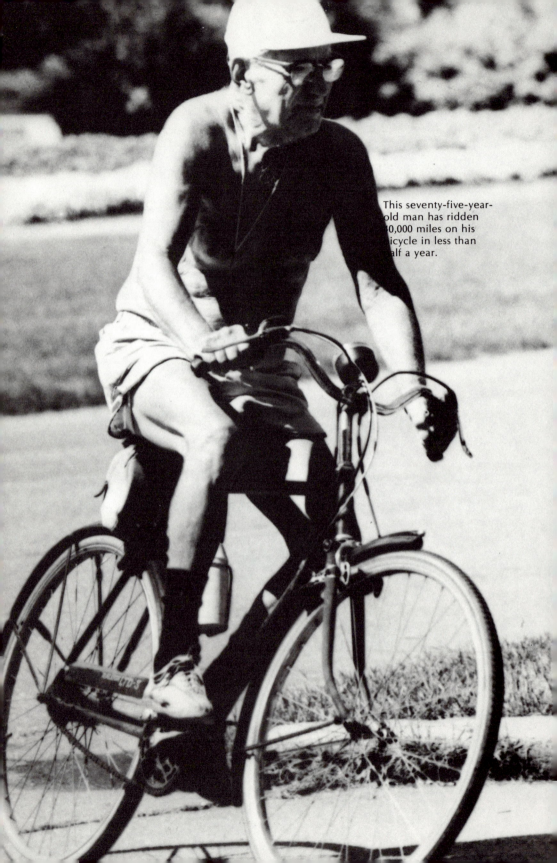

This seventy-five-year-old man has ridden 40,000 miles on his bicycle in less than half a year.

# Chapter Ten

# MAKING OPTIMAL PHYSICAL FITNESS A REALITY: SUMMARY AND CONCLUSIONS

*"Gaining fitness is a process of adapting to stress,
but too much stress leads to injuries and illnesses.
The problem is finding the balance."*

*Dr. George Sheehan*

## MAJOR CONSIDERATIONS IN DESIGNING YOUR EXERCISE PROGRAM

**Although the need for physical activity is universal, no single exercise prescription can serve all individuals.** Created from different molds and varying in so many ways with respect to health status, age, physiological capacity, interests, time availability, and so on, people will invariably fulfill this need through rather diversified patterns of physical activity. **In short, questions concerning "What kinds?", "How much?", and "When?" to exercise are best answered on a personal basis.** The comprehension and appreciation of knowledge pertaining to the nature of physical fitness, exercise guidelines and considerations, and the diverse modes of physical activity previously discussed — together with the information summarized in this final chapter of the text — hopefully will provide each of you with an improved framework for designing your own unique physical activity program.

# 1. PREPARATORY STEPS: FITNESS NEEDS ASSESSMENT AND REALISTIC GOAL SETTING

The initial step in the preparation of an individualized exercise regimen at any stage of life should be the setting of goals that are in line with your fitness needs. Some questions to consider at the start might be: Is there a pressing need to improve aerobic development? Do I seem to lack flexibility in major joints and/or minimal strength-endurance capacities in the locomotive areas of the body? Might I have an obesity problem, or perhaps am I prone to one? The answers to vital questions like these could emanate from: (1) an analysis of your current fitness-related habits; (2) closer observation of your body appearance and the reaction of the locomotive and service networks to everyday physical stress; (3) a physician's advice following medical examination; or (4) actual physical fitness evaluations. Appraisals of the three components of fitness (Chapter 4) point not only to major fitness limitations but provide an objective means for deciding a suitable beginning exercise dosage as well as a baseline for determining the results of your exercise efforts. When no particular weaknesses exist, efforts should be devoted either to maintenance or to further improvement of your current physical fitness status.

Although stated previously, it is worth repeating at this time the idea that all who exercise should devote their efforts toward the following goals:

- **Conditioning of service network (aerobic) processes.**
- **Conditioning within major locomotive areas of the body.**

- **Maintenance or improvement in body leanness.**
- **Psychological rewards such as tension-anxiety release, fun, enjoyment, and relaxation.**
- **Better overall health.**

Evidently, the goals of an exercise program must be realistic and reasonable. Recall the concept of optimal physical fitness and the fact that many uncontrolled forces such as genetic endowment can limit your potential for fitness development. It would be futile for a person with average cardiovascular respiratory efficiency to strive to develop a level of aerobic power requisite to an olympic distance swimmer. Nor should every jogger become capable of completing a 26-mile marathon. **Frustration, physical exhaustion, unhappiness, injury, and illness are risked when you set fitness goals beyond your achievement potential.**

## 2. THE QUESTION OF HOW MUCH EXERCISE TO PERFORM

The determination of a suitable amount of exercise to perform is not to be taken for granted. Dosage, you should remember, is a composite of exercise intensity, duration, and frequency (Chapter 5). Situations exist when dosage (as well as kinds of exercise to perform) should be prescribed by experts or specialists — as do cardiologists and orthopedists for many of their patients. The range in what constitutes suitable dosages for healthy individuals is quite wide, depending, of course, on one's level of physical fitness. The general rule, holding to the principles of readiness, progression, and overload (Chapter 5) is to begin the program with a dosage your body is capable of handling and to increase it only as physiological adaptation is evidenced. To illustrate this critical point, let us consider the predicament of a somewhat sedentary young female whose primary fitness goal is to enhance aerobic endurance to a degree whereby she is capable of jogging (at a slow rate) for thirty minutes without stopping. She might best start with ten-minute jogging workouts (of light intensity that elevate the heart rate to a level no more than 60-70 percent of maximal heart rate) performed three times per week. As time passes and feelings of improvement in stamina are experienced, the duration and frequency of the workouts would gradually be increased. If desired, the intensity of the exercise bouts could also be magnified by elevating the rate or speed of jogging. When the capacity to jog continuously for thirty minutes is accomplished, the young girl could maintain her jogging program without subsequent dosage increments — or with them, if new goals were then set.

The return of your body to its normal resting level of homeostasis following the stress of exercise is critical. Recovery time and, thus, your spacing of workouts depend ultimately on your recovery capacity and the intensity and duration of the exercise bout. Usually, the more strenuous the energy demands of the workout, the longer the time required for the body's return to its normal state of internal equilibrium. Recovery ability does quicken, however, as physical fitness improves. It is not unusual for very fit performers in training for high level athletic competition to engage in several daily workouts spaced only hours apart from one another.

---

# 3. APPROPRIATE PHYSICAL ACTIVITY SELECTION

---

**Three essential requisites for a suitable mode of physical activity include: (1) interest, (2) capability, and (3) practicality.** In complying to a rather basic characteristic of human nature, people will persist in the performance of physical activities they find interesting and satisfying and eventually abandon those they deem unrewarding. Some derive joy from solitary exercise activities such as weight-training and distance swimming or jogging; others might prefer the social atmosphere of aerobic dancing. The competition of sport has excited legions of participants for years and yet fails to excite those of us who tend to be noncompetitive or poorly skilled in athletics.

Obviously, if you are to derive physiological benefits from a particular physical activity, you must have minimal competency

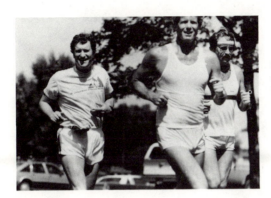

Some people enjoy exercising alone; others with their friends.

to perform it. Wouldn't it be futile for a poorly skilled swimmer, for instance, to construct an interval swimming conditioning program designed to develop aerobic power? Each of you should try to discover one or more physical activities you find rewarding and which you could perform (or would be able to learn) well enough to create adequate physiological demands on your body. **As you approach adulthood, it is strongly advocated that you develop interest, skill, and knowledge in fitness tasks that have "carry-over" value, that is, lend themselves to being performed throughout life.**

The capability requisite for exercise involves not only the skill factor but age and fitness status as well. Almost any mode of exercise would be appropriate for healthy people of all ages, provided dosage is in line with physiological readiness. Certain individuals in excellent health and physical condition are currently performing competitive sports well beyond the age of sixty. Others who recognize their limitations or who have been advised to refrain from the more competitive and demanding physical activities might best pursue exercise programs that incorporate walking, light jogging, swimming, calisthenics, and stretching activities. Golf, for example, is certainly a suitable aerobic endurance activity for an older, less vigorous person; whereas handball, which has an energy expenditure that is five times that of golfing, would be more appropriate for a person with a higher degree of aerobic power.

Lastly, one should be free from any illness or infirmity that might be compounded through the performance of a particular physical activity. Certainly, those of us with orthopedic prob-

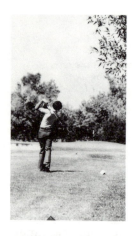 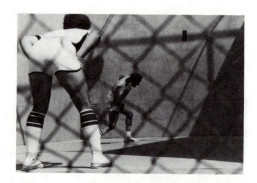

Golf may be a suitable aerobic endurance activity for an older, less vigorous person, while handball would be more appropriate for a person with a higher degree of aerobic power.

lems associated with the feet, ankles, or knees would derive more benefits from the likes of less traumatic non-weight-bearing activities, such as swimming or cycling, rather than from jogging or sports that involve repetitive pounding and jarring of these joints.

Opportunities to participate in almost any type of physical activity desired exist to a greater degree today than ever before.

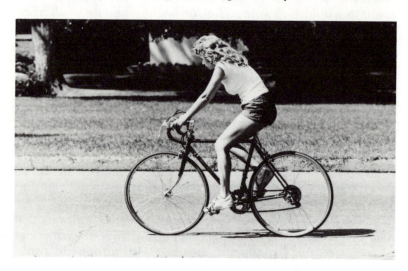

Walking has always been a most popular form of exercise because it is so convenient to perform at any time or place. From time immemorial, males and females of all ages have exercised their bodies through popular sports and active games. Periodically, certain physical activities (such as jogging and cycling) captivate the interest of great numbers of people; only time, however, will determine whether or not they are fads.

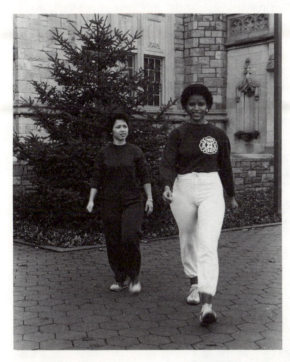

Walking is perhaps the physical activity with the least requisites for participation.

Although sport has withstood the test of time, many of the current popular ones such as skiing, tennis, racketball, golf, sailing, and squash can be expensive to perform on a regular basis. Equipment is costly, and user fees for required facilities can be draining to one's finances. In terms of accessibility, it is fairly easy to arrange a workout for solitary or small group physical activities that require a minimum in the way of facilities and equipment. Team sports including basketball, volleyball, and softball are growing in popularity among our adult population, but necessitate the recruitment of other players and a special area of play. Thus, they cannot always be performed when one desires. **Basic fitness activities including walking, jogging, calisthenics, and rope skipping, on the other hand, require the least requisites for participation in terms of other competitors, movement skills, equipment, and facilities.** In fact, an excellent workout can be derived from these activities at any time of the day that one desires. They can also be performed within groups or alone, in just about any type of indoor or outdoor area including playgrounds, backyards, cellars, rooftops, garages, classrooms, hallways, corridors, and even living rooms. Unfortunately, too many of us find such exercise tasks tedious and unexciting. Exercising while listening to your favorite kind of music, however, might greatly alleviate the boredom and monotony that you experience during the performance of activities such as rope skipping, in-place jogging, calisthenics, weight training, and stretching.

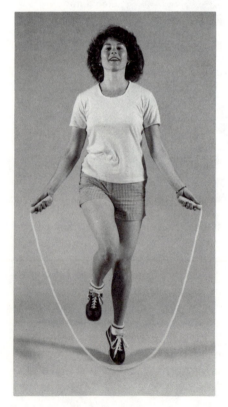

Rope skipping is an excellent basic fitness activity.

Sports and many forms of dance do lend themselves to fitness promotion, but not to the extent of more specific conditioning regimens. Interval training, jogging, circuit training, weight training, and progressive stretching are more systematized, better regulated, and have built-in evaluation systems to indicate fitness progress. Most significant is the fact that exercise-related goals are more likely to be attained because of effective control of dosage progression requisite to physiological adaptations within the body's fitness networks. **The role of general conditioning activities in the enhancement of both safety and performance levels of athletes and dancers is well accepted today.** The movements of sports and dance activities are inherently stressful to the muscles, bones, and joints utilized in their performance — some more so than others. To guard against injury, levels of strength, endurance, and flexibility should be elevated beyond the requirements of the sport or dance performed. For example, a college baseball pitcher or a middle-aged tennis player is exercising the elbow and shoulder areas via the throwing and serving motions. However, the constant repetition of these movement patterns can overtax the soft tissues of the elbow and shoulder. A higher degree of protection from the potential trauma and wear and tear caused by throwing and serving could result from the regular practice of specific progressive resistance and stretching tasks that elevate the strength, endurance, and range of motion within the elbow and shoulder of the performer. In a similar vein, it is also wise to condition the service systems several times per week through typical aerobic activities, thus elevating aerobic power or endurance beyond the levels required by one's sport or dance performance.

## 4. WHEN TO EXERCISE?

The best time of day to exercise is also individually determined. Certain persons operate more effectively in the morning hours, while others function better later in the day. You should attempt to exercise at a time when you feel at your best and when weather and other personal factors permit it.

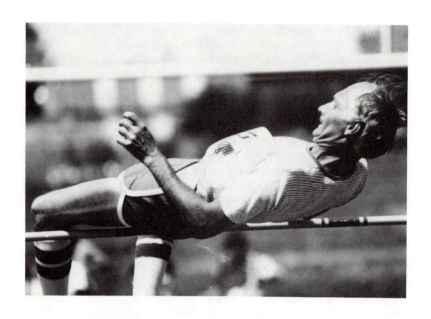

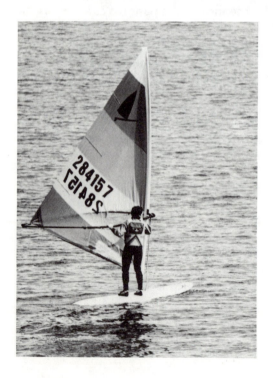

In discussions with them, many students and adult friends have rationalized that they are far to busy to exercise regularly. "With so many daily responsibilities and commitments, how on earth could I appropriate time for physical activity too?" My counterargument is that if you can find the time to eat, read a newspaper, and watch television, then you can certainly re-arrange your priorities to include a 20-30 minute period of exercise in your daily schedule! Others claim that they are too exhausted by day's end to even think about exercise. **It is quite unfortunate that there are so many of you who think this way and who fail to recognize the fact that exercise is an "ener-gizer." That is, it activates the nervous system as well as induces the flow of hormones through the body. Those who exercise regularly have discovered they have more and not less pep and vitality after their daily workout!** And, if you truly find it difficult to perform physical activity during or following a hectic school or work day, there is another alternative. Try to retire somewhat earlier at night and arise an hour or two earlier in the morning for a pre-breakfast workout. Many people are discovering that early morning exercise is both enjoyable and exhilarating and that they can better face daily responsibilities with post-exercise feelings of confidence and freshness.

Because it does arouse the nervous and endocrine systems, one should refrain from strenuous exercise prior to bedtime (to avoid sleep interference). Heavy physical activity after a large meal is also not advocated because it disturbs the digestive processes.

# FINAL THOUGHTS: PATIENCE AND PERSISTENCE

**Initial workouts when beginning a physical conditioning program are always the most difficult and challenging. Feelings of uncertainty, dejection, and/or doubt are not uncommon among neophytes who fail to experience "instant fitness" following the first few encounters with exercise.** While a firm believer and advocate of exercise, the author is a realist as well. He can make no promise of quick, miraculous fitness gains.

Question those who do, and beware of quacks who guarantee remarkable outcomes from a few short periods of exercise! Recall that fitness improvements in service and locomotive organs are best assured by regular participation in **a minimal of three weekly 20-30 minute bouts of exercise.** And even then, do not expect evidence of physiological adaptations to be manifested until after **at least 5-6 weeks of faithful exercise.**

**Be patient, persist, and progress gradually in your exercise efforts. Above all else, enjoy them!** Results from your endeavors will indeed be eventually realized. Slight to moderate discomfort including labored breathing and dry mouth, which are often felt during the early stages of conditioning, dissipate with time. Local (muscle-joint) soreness and stiffness following a workout and periodic regression in exercise performance are other normal expectations that should be anticipated as the body proceeds to adapt to increased energy demands imposed upon it. However, abnormalities such as excessive discomfort or feelings of sickness during exercise or severe persistent pain, stiffness, or soreness, and total body exhaustion following exercise are not to be taken lightly. Such symptoms reflect overstress or incomplete recovery from previous workouts. When they appear, exercise should be curtailed in one or more aspects of dosage and rest provided for full recovery.

Remember that exercise for improvement of aerobic and locomotive efficiency, obesity control, or general health does not necessitate adherence to a rigid physical activity schedule from which one can never deviate. **In fact, variations in exercise routines are not only rewarding and refreshing psychologically but could be physiologically advantageous as well.** Even when the exact same muscles and joints are activated by varying activities, they seem to respond somewhat differently to the particular kind of movements that tax them. Therefore, periodic alternation of patterns of physical activity (rather than the exclusive participation in the same form of it) tend to be less draining to locomotive organs while promoting their recovery to a greater degree.

Lastly, keep in mind that all physiological changes produced via systematic exercise respond rather quickly to inactivity and decreased metabolic demands. **In other words, it will take little time for the sedentary body to lose all those benefits derived through so much effort and time spent in**

**conditioning it.** Once fitness gains are realized, exercise dosage of sufficient levels to maintain them must be performed on a regular year-round basis. **In short, although optimal physical fitness requires a lifetime of effort, it is well worth it!**

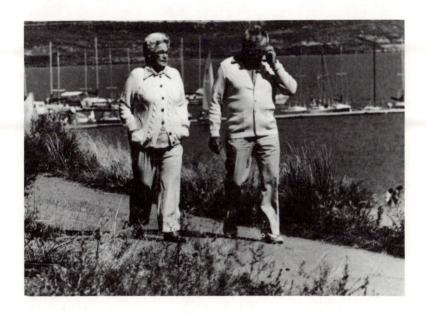

# REFERENCES

Anderson, J. L. *The Yearbook of Sports Medicine.* Chicago: Yearbook Medical Publishers, 1981.

Anderson, Bob. *Stretching.* Bolinas, California: Shelter Publications, 1980.

Banhorn, George. *Food for Fitness.* Mountain View, California: Anderson World Publications, 1975.

Cooper, Kenneth H. *The Aerobics Program for Total Well-Being.* New York: M. Evans, 1982.

Fox, E. L. and D. K. Mathews. *Interval Training: Conditioning for Sports and General Fitness.* Philadelphia: W. B. Saunders Co., 1974.

Fox, E. L. and D. K. Mathews. *The Physiological Basis of Physical Education and Athletics.* Philadelphia: W. B. Saunders Co., 1976.

Johnson, Perry, et. al. *Sport, Exercise, and You.* New York: Holt, Rinehart and Winston, 1975.

Kantzleman, Beth. *Complete Guide to Aerobic Dancing.* New York: Fawcett Books, 1979.

Kash, Frank. *Adult Fitness: Principles and Practice.* Palo Alto, California: Mayfield Publishing Co., 1968.

Katch, F. and W. McArdle. *Nutrition, Weight Control, and Exercise.* Boston: Houghton Mifflin Co., 1977.

Kisselle, L. and K. Mazzeo. *Aerobic Dance: A Way To Fitness.* Denver, Colorado: Morton Publishing Co., 1983.

Klafs, C. and D. Arnheim. *Modern Principles of Athletic Training.* St. Louis: The C. V. Mosby Co., 1977.

Leon, Edie. *Complete Women's Weight Training Guide.* Mountain View, California: Anderson World Publications, 1976.

Logan, G. and W. McKinney. *Anatomic Kinesiology.* Dubuque, Iowa: Wm. C. Brown Co., Publishers, 1977.

Olson, O. C. *Prevention of Injuries: Protecting the Health of the Student Athlete.* Philadelphia: Lea and Febiger Publishers, 1971.

Sacks, Michael. *Psychology of Running.* Champaign, Illinois: Human Kinetics Publishers, 1981.

Schonfeld, David. *Yoga for a Better Life.* Wheaton, Illinois: Theosophical Publishing House, 1980.

Sharkey, Brian. *Physiology and Physical Activity.* New York: Harper and Row Publishers, 1975.

Sharkey, Brian. *Physiology of Fitness.* Champaign, Illinois: Human Kinetics Publishers, 1979.

Smith, Nathan. *Food for Sport.* Palo Alto, California: Bull Publishing Co., 1976.

Sobey, Edwin. *Complete Circuit Training Guide.* Mountain View, California: Anderson World Publishers, 1980.

Sorensen, Jackie. *Aerobic Dancing.* New York: Rawson Wade Publishers, 1979.

Uram, Paul. *Complete Stretching Book.* Mountain View, California: Anderson World Publications, 1980.

U.S. Dept. of Agriculture, U.S. Dept. of Health and Human Services. *Home Garden Bulletin No. 232, "Nutrition And Your Health, Dietary Guidelines For Americans."* February, 1980.

U.S. Dept. of Agriculture. *Food and Your Weight.* Washington, D.C.: U.S. Government Printing Office, 1973.

Vincent, L. M. *The Dancer's Book of Health.* Kansas City: Sheed Andrews and McMeel, Inc., 1978.

Westcott, Wayne. *Strength Fitness: Physiological Principles and Training Techniques.* Boston: Allyn and Bacon, Inc., 1982.

Wilmore, Jack. *Athletic Training and Physical Education: Physiological Principles and Practices of the Conditioning Process.* Boston: Allyn and Bacon, Inc., 1976.

Zohman, Lenore, et. al. *The Cardiologists' Guide to Fitness and Health Through Exercise.* New York: Simon and Schuster Publishers, 1979.

# GLOSSARY

**Acclimatization**
The ability of the body to adapt itself to extreme warm or cold weather conditions.

**Adipose**
Fat tissue. (Adiposecyte is the name of the fat cell).

**Aerobic Dance**
A combination of repetitive dance steps, stretching, and other simple movement routines performed to popular music.

**Aerobic Efficiency**
The operational effectiveness of the service network systems in providing oxygenated blood to working muscles. (Also referred to as cardiovascular-respiratory fitness and service network efficiency.)

**Aerobic Endurance Exercise**
Light to moderate physical activities that do not demand large volumes of oxygenated blood (to working muscles); and thus can be sustained for long time periods.

**Aerobic Exercise**
Exercise that activates the service network to supply adequate oxygen to muscles to sustain their energy production.

**Aerobic Power Exercise**
Strenuous physical activity that demands a larger volume of oxygenated blood for working muscles (per minute).

**Anaerobic Exercise**
Strenuous and short-lived physical activity where the demands for oxygen by working muscles exceeds the service system's capacity to deliver it.

**Anti-Gravity Muscles**
Body muscles that contract automatically to keep weight-bearing joints straight (joint extensors).

**Appetite**
The desire or craving for food.

### Balance Principle
The development of each component of physical fitness as well as an effective, well-rounded exercise program.

### Ballistic Stretch
Stretching movements that involve lunging, jerking, or bouncing.

### Body Leanness
The component of physical fitness characterized by the dominance of lean tissues (as opposed to adipose tissue).

### Calisthenics
Elementary body movements made against gravity; and executed in upright, sitting or lying positions.

### Caloric Balance
See energy balance.

### Caloric Output
See energy expenditure.

### Caloric Intake
See energy intake.

### Cardiovascular-Respiratory Fitness
See aerobic efficiency.

### Circuit Training
Performance of a core of exercise tasks sequentially in three sets and within a designated time period.

### Cool Down
The post exercise period.

### Continuous Exercise
Physical activity performed in a "steady state" (that is with little fluctuation in energy output).

### Core
A group of movement or exercise tasks.

### Cramp
State of involuntary muscle contraction that results in pain and movement incapacitation.

### Creeping Obesity
The gradual accretion of adipose that commences during the early adult years of life.

### Critical Threshold
The minimal exercise heart rate required to cause functional improvements within power mechanisms of the service network.

**Desirable Weight**
An average body weight (in lbs.) based on age, sex, and height.

**Dosage**
The amount of exercise performed in one week.

**Duration**
The time involved in an exercise workout.

**Energy Balance**
Energy Intake equals energy expenditure. (also Caloric Balance)

**Energy Expenditure**
The energy expended or burned by the body over a specific period of time. (e.g. one day) most often expressed in kilocalories. (also Caloric Output).

**Energy Intake**
The total number of kilocalories contained in the food (eaten in one day). (also Caloric Intake).

**Exercise**
The performance of muscular work through popular movement activities. (physical activity)

**Exercise Fuels**
Carbohydrate and fat used in energy production within muscles.

**Fat Body Weight (FBW)**
The number of pounds of fat tissue within the body.

**Flexibility**
The ability of a joint to move through full range of motion.

**Frequency**
The number of exercise work-outs per week.

**Heart Rate**
The number of heart beats per minute. (also called pulse rate).

**Heat Exhaustion**
Temporary state of illness due to exposure to warm weather conditions and sun rays.

**Heat Stroke**
Excessive internal body temperature rise that can cause shock and death; (if not alleviated immediately).

**Homeostasis**
A state of equilibrium or balance throughout internal tissue environs.

**Hunger**
The physiological need for food.

### Hyperventilation
Rapid, deep breathing.

### Hypothermia
Excessive decline or reduction of body temperature.

### Individualized Physical Activity
Physical activity geared to a personal need, interest, and capacity.

### Intensity (exercise)
The degree of exercise stress or demand.

### Interval Physical Activity
Physical activities that involve alternating periods of high and low energy demands. (also intermittent exercise)

### Isokinetics
A form of resistance exercise involving movements from a pre-stretched position and whereby the resistance equals the level of tension created throughout the movement.

### Isometrics
Movements attempted against immovable resistances.

### Kilocalorie (Calorie)
An expression of unit of energy to measure energy production within the body, and energy potential of ingested foods. (it is equal to the amount of heat required to raise a kilogram of water one degree centigrade.)

### Lean Body Weight (LBW)
The number of pounds of lean tissues within the body.

### Locomotive Network
The systems of the body involved in the production of movement; namely the muscles, bones, joints and nerves.

### Locomotive Network Efficiency
The effective means of operation within the varying parts of the locomotive organs.

### Maintenance Principle
Constant exercise dosage required to maintain one's state of physical fitness.

### Maximum Heart Rate
The highest number of times the heart can beat per minute.

### Metabolic Rate (Basal Metabolic Rate)
The degree of total body energy expenditure (at a specific time as expressed in kilocalories).

**Metabolism**
All the complex reactions that are undertaken at the cellular level.

**Muscle Endurance**
The ability of muscle to sustain operations for long time periods.

**Obesity**
A condition in which the body is burdened with excessive adipose tissue.

**Optimal Physical Fitness**
The highest level of personal or individual physical fitness attainable.

**Overeating**
The consumption of more food than the body actually needs.

**Overexercise**
Exercise dosage beyond one's state of readiness.

**Overload**
The progressive upgrading of total metabolic demands, or degree of stress of an exercise task.

**Overweight**
Pounds above desirable weight.

**Nautilus**
An exercise apparatus used in isokinetic training.

**Negative Energy Balance**
Energy expenditure exceeds energy intake (usually resulting in fat weight loss).

**Percent Body Fat**
The percentage of total body weight that is fat.

**Physical Fitness**
A dynamic state of being characterized by three integrated components; body leanness, service network efficiency, and locomotive network efficiency.

**Positive Energy Balance**
Energy intake is greater than energy expenditure (resulting in the storage of energy usually in the form of fat).

**Power**
The ability of a muscle to build up tension quickly (or explosively).

**Progression**
Gradual increments in exercise dosage that are in line with readiness of the exercise performer.

**Pulse Rate**
See heart rate.

**Readiness Principle**
A state of being both physiologically and phychologically capable of handling the demands of exercise.

**Regularity Principle**
Performance of physical activity on a regular or systematic basis (rather than sporadically).

**Regulatory Network**
The systems of the body that control the happenings within the locomotive and service networks.

**Rep**
The number of times a specific exercise task is repeated.

**Second Wind**
Dissipation of (respiratory) discomfort, and a renewed capacity and desire to continue exercise.

**Service Network**
The systems of the body that continuously supply nutrients to and removal of wastes from all its operating parts.

**Service Network Efficiency**
See Aerobic efficiency.

**Set**
The completion of a core of exercise tasks.

**Side Stitch**
Stabbing pain felt on the side and near the bottom of the rib cage during exercise; which can be excrutiating at times but is generally not dangerous.

**Specificity Principle**
The physiological outcome or adaptation resulting from exercise is specific to (totally dependent upon) the particular organs and tissues stressed by that physical activity.

**Stability (bone and joint)**
Capacity of bones and joints to resist the stress of forceful movements.

**Static Stretch**
Holding a stretched position (or posture) for a minimum of 12 seconds.

**Steady State (exercise)**
Physical activity that is sustained or carried out at an even rate (of energy expenditure) for three or more minutes.

**Strength**
The maximum force or tension a muscle can exert on lifting, pushing, or pulling a resistance.

**Target Heart Rate**
The heart rate that one desires to attain during a workout.

**Third Wind**
Feeling of euphoria (or a "high") experienced in long duration aerobic physical activity periods.

**Underweight**
Pounds under or below desirable weight.

**Universal**
A multi-stationed exercise device used in weight training.

**Warm-Up**
Initial phase of an exercise work-out to prepare the body for the more strenuous physical activity to follow.

**Weight Training**
Exercise movements executed against some form of resistive device.

**Work-Out**
An exercise period or bout.

# Appendix

# PHYSICAL ACTIVITY RECORD CHARTS

The basic physical activity charts that follow are included for those of you who desire to keep records of your progress in varying exercise programs that you elect to perform.

# AEROBIC EXERCISE PROGRAM RECORD CHART

Name _____ Class_____

Date Started _____ Date Completed _____

## INSTRUCTIONS

- Determine a suitable exercise intensity based on your desired target heart rate zone, and/or perceived rate of exertion (RPE) for each aerobic workout.
- Calculate your exercise HR (approximately at the half way point of the workout).
- Record it along with your RPE and the duration of the exercise bout in the spaces provided.

| DATE | PHYSICAL ACTIVITY | DURATION | EXERCISE HR | RPE |
|------|-------------------|----------|-------------|-----|
|      |                   |          |             |     |
|      |                   |          |             |     |
|      |                   |          |             |     |
|      |                   |          |             |     |
|      |                   |          |             |     |
|      |                   |          |             |     |
|      |                   |          |             |     |
|      |                   |          |             |     |
|      |                   |          |             |     |
|      |                   |          |             |     |
|      |                   |          |             |     |
|      |                   |          |             |     |

# CIRCUIT TRAINING RECORD CHARTS

Name _____ Class_____

Date Started _____ Date Completed _____

## INSTRUCTIONS

- Select either a pre-constructed or self-designed circuit training program.
- If you desire to perform a self-constructed circuit training regimen, first complete the *Self-Designed Circuit Training Information Chart* below via a testing period. Once accomplished, transfer the data to the *Circuit Training Record Log* that follows.
- Students electing to perform a pre-constructed circuit program can proceed directly to the recording of the required information in the *Circuit Training Record Log.*

## SELF-DESIGNED CIRCUIT TRAINING INFORMATION CHART

TESTING DATES:   ONE_____   TWO_____   THREE_____

| Core Exercise | Test Performance Time | | | | Total Reps | | | | One-Half or Three-Quarter Reps | | | |
|---|---|---|---|---|---|---|---|---|---|---|---|---|
| | Tests: | One | Two | Three | Tests: | One | Two | Three | Tests: | One | Two | Three |
| | | | | | | | | | | | | |
| | | | | | | | | | | | | |
| | | | | | | | | | | | | |
| | | | | | | | | | | | | |
| | | | | | | | | | | | | |
| | | | | | | | | | | | | |
| | | | | | | | | | | | | |
| | | | | | | | | | | | | |
| | | | | | | | | | | | | |

Totals: _____

Total Test Time_____ × Three = _____ Circuit Target Time

# CIRCUIT TRAINING RECORD LOG

| Date | Number of Core Exercises | Circuit Target Time | Time in Completing Circuit | Exercise HR | RPE |
|------|--------------------------|---------------------|----------------------------|-------------|-----|
|      |                          |                     |                            |             |     |
|      |                          |                     |                            |             |     |
|      |                          |                     |                            |             |     |
|      |                          |                     |                            |             |     |
|      |                          |                     |                            |             |     |
|      |                          |                     |                            |             |     |
|      |                          |                     |                            |             |     |
|      |                          |                     |                            |             |     |
|      |                          |                     |                            |             |     |
|      |                          |                     |                            |             |     |
|      |                          |                     |                            |             |     |
|      |                          |                     |                            |             |     |
|      |                          |                     |                            |             |     |
|      |                          |                     |                            |             |     |
|      |                          |                     |                            |             |     |
|      |                          |                     |                            |             |     |
|      |                          |                     |                            |             |     |
|      |                          |                     |                            |             |     |

# CALISTHENIC AND STRETCHING EXERCISE PROGRAM RECORD CHART

Name _____ Class _____

Date Started _____ Date Completed _____

## INSTRUCTIONS

- Select a suitable core of calisthenic and/or stretching exercise tasks to perform.
- Record the number of sets and reps performed for each exercise selected at each workout.

Starting Date _____ Date Completed _____

### CORE OF CALISTHENIC AND STRETCHING EXERCISES

Exercise Tasks

| Workout Date | 1. Sets | Reps | 2. Sets | Reps | 3. Sets | Reps | 4. Sets | Reps | 5. Sets | Reps | 6. Sets | Reps | 7. Sets | Reps | 8. Sets | Reps | 9. Sets | Reps | 10. Sets | Reps | 11. Sets | Reps | 12. Sets | Reps |
|---|---|---|---|---|---|---|---|---|---|---|---|---|---|---|---|---|---|---|---|---|---|---|---|---|
|  |  |  |  |  |  |  |  |  |  |  |  |  |  |  |  |  |  |  |  |  |  |  |  |  |
|  |  |  |  |  |  |  |  |  |  |  |  |  |  |  |  |  |  |  |  |  |  |  |  |  |
|  |  |  |  |  |  |  |  |  |  |  |  |  |  |  |  |  |  |  |  |  |  |  |  |  |
|  |  |  |  |  |  |  |  |  |  |  |  |  |  |  |  |  |  |  |  |  |  |  |  |  |
|  |  |  |  |  |  |  |  |  |  |  |  |  |  |  |  |  |  |  |  |  |  |  |  |  |
|  |  |  |  |  |  |  |  |  |  |  |  |  |  |  |  |  |  |  |  |  |  |  |  |  |
|  |  |  |  |  |  |  |  |  |  |  |  |  |  |  |  |  |  |  |  |  |  |  |  |  |
|  |  |  |  |  |  |  |  |  |  |  |  |  |  |  |  |  |  |  |  |  |  |  |  |  |

# WEIGHT TRAINING RECORD CHARTS

Name _____ Class _____

Date Started _____ Date Completed _____

## INSTRUCTIONS

- Depending on your weight training objectives, follow either **Prescription A** (maximum strength development) or **Prescription B** (maximum endurance development) (See Table 7.3, page 125).
- Increase weight resistance when predetermined reps and sets are accomplished with the previous weight.
- Record resistance changes (new resistances) and the dates they take effect in the *Weight Training Resistance Record Chart* below.
- Record all weight training information in the *Weight Training Workout Logbook* that follows.

## WEIGHT TRAINING RESISTANCE RECORD CHART

| Weight Training Exercise Core | Date: | Starting Resistance | Date: | New Resistance | Date: | New Resistance |
|---|---|---|---|---|---|---|
| | | | | | | |
| | | | | | | |
| | | | | | | |
| | | | | | | |
| | | | | | | |
| | | | | | | |
| | | | | | | |
| | | | | | | |

# WEIGHT TRAINING WORKOUT LOGBOOK

EXERCISE TASK: _____

| Date | Resistance | Repetitions | | |
|------|-----------|-------------|-----------|-----------|
| | | **First Set** | **Second Set** | **Third Set** |
| | | | | |
| | | | | |
| | | | | |
| | | | | |
| | | | | |
| | | | | |
| | | | | |
| | | | | |
| | | | | |

EXERCISE TASK: _____

| Date | Resistance | Repetitions | | |
|------|-----------|-------------|-----------|-----------|
| | | **First Set** | **Second Set** | **Third Set** |
| | | | | |
| | | | | |
| | | | | |
| | | | | |
| | | | | |
| | | | | |
| | | | | |
| | | | | |
| | | | | |

# WEIGHT TRAINING WORKOUT LOGBOOK

EXERCISE TASK: _____

| Date | Resistance | Repetitions | | |
|------|------------|-----------|------------|-----------|
|      |            | First Set | Second Set | Third Set |
|      |            |           |            |           |
|      |            |           |            |           |
|      |            |           |            |           |
|      |            |           |            |           |
|      |            |           |            |           |
|      |            |           |            |           |
|      |            |           |            |           |
|      |            |           |            |           |
|      |            |           |            |           |
|      |            |           |            |           |

EXERCISE TASK: _____

| Date | Resistance | Repetitions | | |
|------|------------|-----------|------------|-----------|
|      |            | First Set | Second Set | Third Set |
|      |            |           |            |           |
|      |            |           |            |           |
|      |            |           |            |           |
|      |            |           |            |           |
|      |            |           |            |           |
|      |            |           |            |           |
|      |            |           |            |           |
|      |            |           |            |           |
|      |            |           |            |           |
|      |            |           |            |           |

# WEIGHT TRAINING WORKOUT LOGBOOK

EXERCISE TASK: _____

| Date | Resistance | Repetitions | | |
|------|------------|-------------|---|---|
| | | First Set | Second Set | Third Set |
| | | | | |
| | | | | |
| | | | | |
| | | | | |
| | | | | |
| | | | | |
| | | | | |
| | | | | |
| | | | | |
| | | | | |

EXERCISE TASK: _____

| Date | Resistance | Repetitions | | |
|------|------------|-------------|---|---|
| | | First Set | Second Set | Third Set |
| | | | | |
| | | | | |
| | | | | |
| | | | | |
| | | | | |
| | | | | |
| | | | | |
| | | | | |
| | | | | |

# WEIGHT TRAINING WORKOUT LOGBOOK

EXERCISE TASK: _____

| Date | Resistance | Repetitions | | |
|------|------------|-------------|------|------|
| | | **First Set** | **Second Set** | **Third Set** |
| | | | | |
| | | | | |
| | | | | |
| | | | | |
| | | | | |
| | | | | |
| | | | | |
| | | | | |
| | | | | |
| | | | | |

EXERCISE TASK: _____

| Date | Resistance | Repetitions | | |
|------|------------|-------------|------|------|
| | | **First Set** | **Second Set** | **Third Set** |
| | | | | |
| | | | | |
| | | | | |
| | | | | |
| | | | | |
| | | | | |
| | | | | |
| | | | | |
| | | | | |
| | | | | |

# WEIGHT TRAINING WORKOUT LOGBOOK

EXERCISE TASK: _____

| Date | Resistance | Repetitions | | |
| | | First Set | Second Set | Third Set |
| --- | --- | --- | --- | --- |
| | | | | |
| | | | | |
| | | | | |
| | | | | |
| | | | | |
| | | | | |
| | | | | |
| | | | | |
| | | | | |
| | | | | |

EXERCISE TASK: _____

| Date | Resistance | Repetitions | | |
| | | First Set | Second Set | Third Set |
| --- | --- | --- | --- | --- |
| | | | | |
| | | | | |
| | | | | |
| | | | | |
| | | | | |
| | | | | |
| | | | | |
| | | | | |
| | | | | |
| | | | | |

# WEIGHT TRAINING WORKOUT LOGBOOK

EXERCISE TASK: _____

| Date | Resistance | Repetitions | | |
| --- | --- | --- | --- | --- |
| | | First Set | Second Set | Third Set |
| | | | | |
| | | | | |
| | | | | |
| | | | | |
| | | | | |
| | | | | |
| | | | | |
| | | | | |
| | | | | |
| | | | | |

EXERCISE TASK: _____

| Date | Resistance | Repetitions | | |
| --- | --- | --- | --- | --- |
| | | First Set | Second Set | Third Set |
| | | | | |
| | | | | |
| | | | | |
| | | | | |
| | | | | |
| | | | | |
| | | | | |
| | | | | |
| | | | | |
| | | | | |

# INDEX